EVERY 'BODY' CAN

THE PROFOUND CHARACTER EVOLUTION FUELLED BY EXERCISE

ADRIAN REDMAN

Contents

For Patsy, the one who believed in me. She saw something in me that I couldn't see in myself at the time.

For the reader, I hope my words not only inspire you, but help you to become everything you are capable of being.

Introduction

As humans, we are wired for movement. Some of us move out of joy, others out of necessity. But for many, there is neither the requirement nor the motivation to move at all. To be physically active by choice, our mind must be in a certain state – one that understands the value of movement and is willing to act on that understanding. And that's not always easy.

Our mindset plays a massive role in our approach to physical activity. And in return, physical activity offers countless benefits – many of which go far beyond the body. This book explores that relationship in depth. Not to win you over to my way of thinking, but to get you thinking. I want the true extent of exercise's power to be common knowledge – because its effects exist whether we acknowledge them or not.

A brief reflection.

For as long as I can remember, exercise has been a part of my life. From athletics in primary school to football and cricket in secondary, and eventually to boxing – it's always been there. I've learned a great deal about myself through movement, but it's through coaching others that I've learned the most. Patterns emerged. I wanted to know if those patterns were universal – if what I observed in one person could apply to every 'body'.

Years of training myself and coaching others led me to a belief: although most societies agree that exercise is important, its true value is still understated. I'm still learning – through every session, every conversation, every 'body' I meet. Whether I'm right or wrong, I stay curious. And it's through curiosity that I gain insight.

I remember being captivated as a child by the **Rocky** films. Physical struggle as a symbol of mental strength. At the time, I didn't fully understand the message – but I felt it. Inspired, I began doing push-ups and sit-ups in the mornings, sprinting up and down the stairs in my house, chasing some undefined idea of improvement. I was around seven years old. I became competitive. If someone was fast, I wanted to be faster. If I lost, I wasn't broken – I just knew I had to improve.

Even outside of sport, this attitude showed up. I remember a spelling test in year 6 – 15 words, I got 14 right. It was the best result in the class that week. My mum was over the moon. But I was disappointed. I wanted more. That drive was the same feeling I got when I trained. Looking back, it was never really about the spelling test or the race. It was about who I was becoming. Maybe **Rocky** didn't create that hunger – maybe it just revealed something that was already there.

At a young age, exercise gave me a sense of control. If I wanted better results, I had to work for them. I applied that same thinking to my schoolwork. One week after my 14/15, I scored a perfect 15/15. It happened to be my birthday. Still one of my favourites.

I used to watch my dad go jogging, but I hated running myself. I did it out of necessity. But over time, I've come to embrace it – not because I suddenly love it, but because I understand the privilege of adversity. There's value in doing the things you hate. Because if you can do what you don't like, and do it consistently, that strengthens your character. Life will take you to dark places. But if you've already pushed yourself into those uncomfortable spaces – on purpose – then when life does it for you, it's familiar territory.

Choose adversity.

CHAPTER 1

The Origins of Exercise

"Even when all is known, the care of a man is not yet complete, because eating alone will not keep a man well; he must also take exercise. For food and exercise, while possessing opposite qualities, yet work together to provide health."
- Hippocrates

It's widely accepted that human physical activity began as a necessity. Our earliest ancestors had to be physically fit to survive – whether that meant hunting for food, escaping predators, or engaging in conflict. Movement wasn't optional; it was life or death.

Hunter-gatherer culture

Hunter-gatherers existed for nearly two million years and still exist in remote parts of the world today – like the Hadza people in northern Tanzania. The demands placed on their bodies were enormous. According to **The American Journal of Medicine,** hunter-gatherers typically walked 6-16 kilometers (about twice the height of Mount Everest) per day, burning between 800 and 1200 kilocalories (about 96000 minutes of running) daily – about five times more than the average adult in modern America.

the men hunted and fished. The women foraged for vegetation. Both roles were physically intense. But survival through physicality didn't stop there – they built shelters, collected firewood, carried children over long distances. Their range of motion and output was like that of modern-day cross-trainers. But there was no structured exercise routine. Their daily life was exercise.

Ancient China - "Exercise is medicine"

China's long history of physical practice – most famously, Kung Fu – dates back over 4,000 years. Originally developed as a method of self-defense, kung fu evolved into a discipline of both body and mind. Every movement was designed to beat an opponent. But it was about more than just winning and losing – it was about life or death. Kung Fu techniques were used by the Chinese to protect themselves from wild animals when hunting. And these techniques were also implemented into military training.

To the Chinese, inactivity was a form of poison. Physical fitness was considered essential not just for strength, but for disease prevention. They held physical activity on the same level of importance as their herbal medicines. Kung Fu wasn't just about fighting; it was a way to test and strengthen the mind. To endure physical extremes and remain calm in the face of chaos – that was the ultimate goal. A strong body, they believed, created a strong mind.

The Roman Empire

No discussion of physical culture is complete without the Roman Empire – a sovereign state whose reign lasted many centuries. Known for its power, strategy, and dominance, Rome owed much of its success to its physically conditioned military. Physical activity was a cornerstone of Roman life – not just for soldiers, but for citizens too. You could be drafted into the army as young as 16 or as late as 40, so there was incentive to stay fit.

According to **The History of Fitness** by Lance C. Dalleck and Len Kravitz, The Roman population had the highest physical fitness condition during the time of the Empire's conquest and expansion.

A lot of the success enjoyed by the Roman Empire can be attributed to the strength of its army. And the strength of its army was largely down to the ways it prepared - intense, tough training.

Ironically, one of the reasons for the Empire's eventual collapse was a decline in that very fitness. As wealth and materialism grew, the population focused more on entertainment. Physical condition took a back seat – and the military suffered for it.

From Necessity to Leisure

As human intellect evolved, so did technology – and with it, convenience. We began creating tools and systems that allowed us to survive with less physical effort. Farming replaced hunting. Eventually, technology replaced farming. But the body hasn't forgotten. We are still wired to move. Even without necessity, the desire remains.

Agriculture: The Beginning of Change

About 12,000 years ago, humans began growing their own food and domesticating animals. Hunting and gathering was no longer a necessity. Our ancestors were now growing a variety of crops such as peas, grains, and wheats, while also herding wild animals. Farming was still physical, but far less demanding than hunting. Over time, fewer individuals needed to farm to feed the population. Eventually, agriculture became a full-time industry – and physical activity in that sense became less of a shared experience.

In today's world, despite farming being big business (responsible for the employment of roughly a billion people worldwide), it is in decline. There is a decreasing trend in the number of farmers on the planet. With a collective increased consumption of processed foods, and the involvement of mass production, it is clear to see why. Today, most of us have no physical role in sourcing our meals. Hunting, gathering, and fishing, are hobbies now, not survival tactics.

Sparta: Fitness as Culture

Sparta is one of the clearest examples of a society that prized physical fitness above nearly everything else. At that time in Greece, there were shared cultural values that were embraced. But the Spartans pushed away some of those "norms" for the sake of physical fitness. Because in Sparta, sport was culture. The women of Sparta stood out; they were different from women elsewhere. It was common for young Spartan girls to participate in several sports at an early age. Their intense physical training continued into adulthood. And for this reason, they had an exceptional physical condition. The collective obsession with health in this region was the driving force behind such discipline.

It was believed in Sparta that the fittest women produced the healthiest offspring – which was the goal. Therefore, a lot of emphasis was placed on making the women as fit as they could be. Unlike other regions of Greece, Spartan women married later – in their late teens. Because it was believed that they would have a healthier pregnancy. They also ate well and trained as hard as the Spartan men. The fascination with producing fit, healthy offspring was taken to the extent of men sharing their wives. If a woman had already produced a healthy child, in the minds of the Spartans, there was a high probability she would repeat that. These choices were not taboo – they were endorsed by the state.

The Olympic games

The first Olympic games were held in Olympia in 776 BCE, created to honour Zeus – king of the Greek Gods. In its early stages, the games featured competitions such as wrestling, running, and chariot racing. These contests reflected the competitive spirit, and physical excellence that was celebrated in Ancient Greek culture. Despite frequent conflict between city-states, the games fostered unity. It was held every four years, featuring participants from different cities across Greece.

Unfortunately, the games were abolished by the Romans in 393 CE. For centuries it was nothing more than a thing of the past. But in 1896, in Athens, the competition was eventually brought back – giving birth to the modern games we know today.

Exercise as punishment

Despite being beneficial, exercise can usually come with some sort of pain. If that pain is without good purpose, we humans will struggle to endure it mentally. This is the reason why historically – and in some instances currently – exercise has been used to inflict punishment. Sir William Cubitt; born 1785, was an English engineer. He is the inventor of the treadmill, which around the time of its creation in 1817 was also referred to as a treadwheel. The initial purpose of the treadmill was to serve as a form of punishment for prisoners, with the intention of lessening the use of the death penalty (yes, even in punishment, exercise still has its benefits). The treadmill punishment was so severe that some prisoners during the 19th century would at times, have to walk on it for up to 6 hours a day. The thought process behind making the treadmill a punishment was that it was seen as pointless, meaning the prisoners would suffer mentally. Consider the contrast with modern times! It wasn't until the late 20th century that the perspective of the treadmill had changed. By that time – because of the jogging revolution – it was being used as a means of gaining fitness. The treadmill is just one example of exercise being used as punishment; not only across England, but in many parts of the world. For example; the 13th Amendment of the Constitution, in the United States allows penal behaviour. The 13th Amendment prohibits slavery 'except as a punishment for a crime whereof the party shall have been duly convicted.'

In some West African cultures, there is a popular method amongst parents when punishing their misbehaving children. 'The frog jump' - squatting, then jumping whilst holding your ears with both hands. This was one of the most dreaded punishments because the parents didn't set a particular number of reps to do, nor did they present a time limit. This same method was also applicable for another West African punishment – 'the invisible chair'. This is what some of us may refer to as a 'wall sit'.

During her time as secretary of state for education (England), Nicky Morgan; in 2014 barred schools from using exercise as a form of correctional behaviour. Using exercise as a punishment was a method introduced by Morgan's predecessor; Michael Gove. Gove saw himself as a traditionalist and was against modern methods of teaching. He felt that stern methods of punishment were an effective way to create more order in the classroom, improving the standard of education. From his perspective, extra physical activity could only be beneficial. Discipline, fitness, improved concentration, and potentially improved academic performance, are amongst these perceived benefits. But many saw the reasons for push-back against Gove's ideas as valid. Parents, teachers, and even athletes – Paula Radcliffe being one of – were rallying against the use of exercise as punishment in schools.

Considering how exercise was once used, and in some instances still is used as punishment, we should understand why it takes such motivation and discipline to incorporate it consistently. Our relationship with physical activity is complex. In its deepest roots, our association with exercise is out of necessity or punishment. Doing it out of choice is somewhat alien to our nature, which is why at times it may feel as though it is too much of a demand. One argument brought forward to oppose Gove's stance was that; using exercise in this way may make students view all physical activity from a negative lens, going forward. If their introduction to physical activity is a negative one, that will be the theme of the relationship they have with it. And if exercise is as beneficial as we say, we should want to incentivise students to immerse themselves long term.

The power of purpose is in our ability to tolerate pain for its sake.

CHAPTER 2

Gender Bias in the World of Fitness

On the surface, we can point to how women from many societies historically have been treated 'fairly' – compared to men – in the world of exercise. The women of Sparta were able to compete in the same sports as the men. And so were women across several African and Native American tribes. In Ancient Rome, exercise was a cultural practice. The earliest Greek athletic competitions didn't include any women; however, it was only inclusive to young men of higher classes – therefore men alike were excluded. And although the first official Olympic games in 1896 didn't include any women, the very next competition four years later hosted 22 female competitors (out of 997 total athletes). But was the low percentage of female competitors due to sexism, or was it simply preference? To argue in favour of the latter; when we examine the work world, the jobs commonly deemed as being more physically demanding are dominated by males, despite equal opportunity for the positions. Therefore, it may be assumed that overall, men may be drawn more to physical activity than women.

As primary caregivers, women of the family usually spend the most time with the infants. This occupies their day. As well as time consuming; child-rearing can be physically and mentally draining, potentially preventing mothers from seeking unnecessary additional activity outside of the home. According to Women's Health Mag; a recent study by Asics' determined that 54% of women in the UK were discontinuing exercise - for reasons such as; lacking self-confidence, a lack of time, and not feeling 'sporty' enough.

In America, the introduction of 'Title IX' (1972) – Civil Rights Act – ensured society recognised women's right to participate in sport on an equal level to men. Despite this, men still outnumber women in sports in the US, while boys significantly outnumber girls. Presented with these facts; it can be easy to reduce it to preference, but there are many ways that these same facts can point towards sexism. A study found that 30% of parents felt that sport was vital for their daughters, whereas 41% felt sport was vital for their sons. With boys outnumbering girls; this could be due to the parents being more inclined to encourage their sons to participate in physical activity, than they are to encourage their daughters. The reasons for the parents doing so could vary, but nevertheless, the outcome is the same. Some females, especially young girls express that they are self-conscious about their bodies. Fearing judgement – due to standards set by society – they avoid scenarios where their body could be a point of focus.

Tragedy to triumph

A friend of mine, Grace, was no stranger to a compliment from me. I admired her commitment, and her discipline, relating to fitness. In some ways she reminded me of myself. Quite often, she seemed to enjoy treats on the sweeter side, like me. But she managed to maintain her figure with ease. I say with ease, not because it doesn't require hard work (it certainly does), but because that hard work became a normality. Fitness became such a fixture in her life, so much so she created a business around it. Her company – Agora Health – was made with the understanding that when it comes to well-being, women have vastly different needs to those of men. Not to mention the complexities of those needs for individual women. Many factors led Grace to the conclusion that a 360 approach towards the well-being of women was the best option. The main reason for her starting Agora Health was due to fitness related restrictions of her own; which were specific to being a woman. Grace was diagnosed with fibroids – which like many women, had an immense physical impact on her. With her weight fluctuating incessantly, she was anxious about her body image. This was something women have experienced throughout history, partly due to the beauty standards portrayed in various forms of media.

Grace experienced her first menstrual cycle at a very young age. The shift in her hormonal balance had a telling effect as she rapidly gained weight. As a ten-year-old experiencing these sudden changes, she confronted it with exercise. Body dysmorphia is something that she had battled at an earlier age. Unaware of it for the most part, but through deep introspection, she was able to realise the issue. "All those years of hormonal imbalance, there was no support from the medical system. I felt very alone in my health journey. Even my trainers couldn't understand how distressed my body was, and the pain I was in. There were months where my only achievement was walking." It wasn't until sixteen years old that she found coaches who provided exercise routines that were specific to her needs. She says this is what led to her falling in love with movement. Despite this, Grace has still encountered trainers in recent years who she believes had preconceived biases towards her, simply because she's a woman. She believed they would often go easy on her; changing their approach, disbelieving she would have certain capabilities. This is something, undoubtedly, many women encounter in the world of fitness. Like many others I've spoken to, Grace stated that exercise helps to ease her period pains; giving her more energy and reducing the feeling of lethargy. It was recently brought to my attention that the monthly cycle, beyond the actual menstruation period, has a significant impact in the ways a woman can work-out. Many women say that during heavy bleeding it would be their preference to refrain from exercise altogether – for one reason or another. And during light bleeding, the preference being some form of light exercise.

- Follicular phase – roughly 7-10 days.

The follicular phase is the longest phase of the menstrual cycle; it overlaps and ensues menstruation. This is the phase where many women feel most energised, and somewhat happier. Due to feeling stronger, and having increased energy levels, this is a good time for women to take their training up a notch and really push themselves. Some recommended exercises for this phase are; swimming, running/cardio.

- Ovulation – roughly 2-4 days.

Following the follicular phase, comes ovulation. Short, but a relatively similar feeling to the follicular – although there may be a difference in mood. Some women may feel discomfort; such as cramps or abdominal pains, but according to many women, they are still able to work-out as they see fit. Recommended exercises; cycling/cardio, cross-fit/boot-camp, HIIT (high intensity interval training).

- Luteal phase – roughly 10-14 days.

This phase is home to 'PMS' (premenstrual syndrome) – this phase comes before menstruation begins again. This is a time where energy levels are generally depleted, and many women report feeling less strength. It is also said that some women might gain up to as much as 5lbs (2.27kg) during this time, while others don't notice any weight gain or bloating at all. However, due to the reduction in energy, this may be a good time for those women who still experience a menstrual cycle to reduce the intensity in their workouts. Understanding the cycle and how it works may prevent women from feeling discouraged to exercise; because not only are they aware of why they may lack energy at times (thus lacking motivation), male trainers would also be aware of this and could tailor a program specific to the woman in question. Recommended exercises; strength training, low incline walking, yoga/pilates.

At the beginning, and end of these 3 phases is the menstrual phase. This is where the period starts and finishes. During this stage, it is recommended that women participate in light, low impact activities. Recommended exercises; yin yoga, mat pilates, walking, foam-rolling.

Although physical fitness can make women prouder of their body image – giving them confidence; Grace feels this could also be an issue. "What I will say is that I think there is a lot of pressure in the fitness industry; given the constant new trends, or body shapes to attain. And this makes us lose sight of why we initially started – which was to align with our health and improve our lives."

Queens of fitness

History boasts many women who were celebrated for their contributions and accomplishments in the world of exercise. Laverie Vallee aka Charmion, was somewhat of a pioneer. Born in 1875 in California, Charmion was raised in a period where it was taboo for women to flaunt their body in a revealing, flamboyant manner. Vallee was a 'strong-woman' - a woman that competed in strength competitions, and/or performed at shows demonstrating her strength. Although plenty of females performed acrobatics; what separated Vallee, aka Charmion was her brave, on stage stripping. She was the first of her kind, therefore she drew mainstream attention. This was at a time when performances like hers were restricted to 'less classy' crowds. During her time – in the late 1800s and early 1900s – it was common for women, and men alike, to exercise wearing full Victorian styled attire. The men would wear full suits (though there was much more variation in their workout gear), and the women wore long dresses.

There were exceptions depending on the sport and the practicality of the attire i.e. swimming or acrobatics. But for the most part, gym-wear was concealing and unexpressive. For women; the dresses were uncomfortable due to the heavy materials, and they limited movement because of the tight design. This gave more power to the symbolism of Charmion's performances by the way she would walk on stage and throw off these uncomfortable garments, stripping down to the more athletic attire in which she performed. Deemed by many as impressive, her physique came from weightlifting and her participation in various sports such as wrestling. Of this she was proud, and she made it known by the way she would show it off – mesmerising crowds. Constantly posing and flexing her muscles; she attracted nationwide attention, eventually touring the US and becoming a superstar. Her style was embraced by the masses, and her rise to fame was inevitable. Performing in major cities, notably New York, she was continually praised for her physique. The newspapers spoke glowingly in the many articles dedicated to her. One article in 1909, read; "She is a type of remarkably developed womanhood. The likes of which probably hasn't been seen since the Roman days." Not every nation met her performances with a keenness - she was forbidden to perform in Germany. But despite this; the positive support for Laverie Vallee, 'Charmion', was overwhelming. She used her fame to promote female health through physical fitness, and even commercialised postcards and pins with her image – posing in ways that highlighted her tremendous physique. Charmion's style was unique for women of that time, but it wasn't unique overall, because some men did similar performances.

So, it begs the question; is her rise to fame (due to the uniqueness of her performances as a woman), proof of biases in the world of fitness that may have existed? Why was it not normal for women to flaunt the results of their physical training, as it was for men? Was this due to the oppression by their male counterparts, or was this simply due to women not being interested in such things? If the latter, was this lack of interest socially constructed; maybe due to the pressure of living up to a particular image? For example, historical images such as 'Venus de Milo' of Ancient Greece; a statue of the goddess Aphrodite – representing beauty and love. We can speculate on the possible reasons behind these gender differences, but it doesn't change the fact that these differences exist(ed).

Jack Lalane, labelled as 'the Godfather of Fitness', is credited for revolutionising the fitness industry. It is widely reported that he introduced weight training and nutrition to the mainstream audience. Lalane is the inventor of many exercise machines; some still being used today. And in 1936 he opened the first ever health and fitness club in the United States. Jack Lalane hosted his own television show that aired for over thirty years on American television. This show – The Jack Lalane Show – received much praise, particularly for being innovative. One of its programs (in the 1950s) was aimed specifically towards women. The wife of Jack; Elaine Lalane, is dubbed 'the First Lady of Physical Fitness'. She has spent decades of her life teaching fitness and health to people of all ages. At the time of this book's publishing, she is 98 years old – and despite her age, she still starts her day with a workout. This workout includes core building exercises such as; full body push-ups, sit ups, and an incline walk. It is no surprise that over the years, Elaine managed to maintain her muscle mass and figure. It is fair to suggest that Mrs. Lalane has also encountered situations – exclusive to women – that may be considered as obstacles. She has birthed three children; and with that, she managed the physical, mental, and social demands. Women like Elaine are not proof of non-existent biases and sexism towards women within the fitness world. Instead, they would be proof that women can thrive, despite those obstacles.

Singer and author, Frankie Bridge, has openly discussed her personal mental health struggles. The way she overcame that battle was through physical fitness, and she created her own fitness and wellness program as a means of helping others in the same way. She spoke about having to adjust her fitness routine since becoming a mother, but she enjoys every moment of it. Whether or not the masses agree with the idea of gender biases within the fitness world, it is wonderful to see so many women – historically and presently – from; Betty Weilder and Val Njord, to the likes of Tammy Hembrow and Paige Hathaway, thriving. They are being recognised and praised for their work and bodies in the same ways that men are.

Is praise and recognition enough? There is still a notable pay gap between men and women in sports. I am not here to argue whether that is due to sexism, or due to a lack of popularity in women's sport (less popularity meaning less income). Rather, I am here to point out that the pay gap exists. And this could be one of the driving factors behind why girls/ women have less desire to participate in sport, when compared to the participation of boys/men.

CHAPTER 3

Mind and body, body and mind

It's mental how the physical starts and ends with the mind. If you want to improve your body; work on the mind. If you want to improve your mind; work on the body. The two, improve your life. Physical adversity is mental adversity, and it is through mental adversity that character is built. Character dictates outcome, and outcome is rationalised by maturity. Yes, it's true that our experiences shape us, but we are in control of our own experiences. What I'm saying is we can use physical activity to shape the outcome of our lives.

"What we mean by mind, is simply that which perceives, thinks, feels, wills, and desires." - Sir William Hamilton

In his book 'Your mind and how to use it', William Walker Atkinson describes the above quote as "inadequate and circular in nature" but admits that there is no other way around it. "This is unavoidable... mind can be defined only by reference to its own processes."

To describe the mind would be to describe its functions. Our mind is responsible for every thought or every feeling we interpret. Therefore, everything in our reality is the consequence of a thought. Meaning; to some degree, our immediate outcomes may be our responsibility. And if that be the case, we must be more deliberate in our thoughts to navigate a particular outcome.

"Healthy body, healthy mind". It is obvious on the surface, but the two have a much deeper connection. Several studies show how improving your physical condition can aid cognitive function and mental well-being. For such a fascinating correlation, it's not widely noted. Of course, without deep thought we may all be able to name several ways in which the two interlink. But once we explore it on a deeper level; we realise the profundity of the connection. Being that the brain is the most metabolically demanding organ in the body, improving blood flow will improve cognitive function. Exercise does exactly this; it improves blood flow to the brain. And when you exercise, your body triggers the release of a chemical called endorphins - feel good transmitters. According to Debra Fulghum Bruce, PhD; endorphins trigger a euphoric feeling similar to that of morphine, and they also diminish the perception of pain. Upon release, the endorphins attach to neuron receptors which are the same receptors that bind some pain medicines.

Exercise in school

Aside from the disadvantages previously expressed – relating to punishment – some have argued that regular exercise/sport in school isn't ideal for other reasons. One of those reasons being unfriendly competition. Competition may cause students to lose sight of the actual purpose; and instead, they end up focusing only on being better than each other. And with the focus being on competition, shame could become a factor. By nature, some of us are less athletic than others; therefore, a clear difference in athletic ability

– when engaging in group exercise – will surface. Due to this, it is natural for some to feel ashamed, thus discouraged. It may cause insecurities and even lead to teasing, but objectively speaking, the advantages for exercise in schools outweighs the potential disadvantages. And those advantages for pupils are beyond physical.

Author John Ratey in his book 'Spark', wrote about an interesting study that took place in Naperville, Illinois (US). This study was groundbreaking as it produced findings to support the claim that exercise in school, essentially makes pupils perform better academically. Back in 1990, Junior High teacher Phil Lawler, was set on introducing more efficient physical exercise in schools. His intention was to improve the overall health of the students. Lawler believed that if they practiced a health positive lifestyle during school years, their habits would last a lifetime. To support his ideas, he introduced what was considered high-tech equipment into schools. While attending a conference, Lawler noticed a heart rate monitor mixed in with some other sports equipment. He admits to stealing it. Like the Robin Hood of fitness, he began using the monitor to track and compare the fitness progression of his physical education students in Junior High.

Since 1992, Naperville Central High School (NCHS) had been using heart rate monitors during physical education for the purposes suggested by Lawler. But in 2003, the level of poor reading skills among students, and a degree of curiosity from a man named Paul Zientarski, led to the heart rate monitors serving a greater purpose.

'Zero-hour PE' was an experiment introduced at Naperville Central High School. Conducted by a group of P.E teachers; the idea of this experiment was to see if there could be some improvement in reading ability and literary results if an intense workout was carried out prior to any academic work. Neil Duncan was the teacher for the first experiment. He took a controlled group of students and had them run around a track. To legitimise the experiment, the controlled group' workout had to be at an intensity higher than any workout carried out by all others at the school. The plan was to have them working at between 80 and 90% of their maximum heart rate (measured using the

monitors). Even the slower students were working at the desired rate because regardless of the time taken to complete the laps, they were still pushing themselves. No surprise to the teachers at NCHS; the controlled group of students showed a 17% improvement in reading and comprehension by the end of the semester. The uncontrolled group showed an increase of just 10% – this was after having the privilege of 'sleeping in' and just doing regular P.E. The conclusion was that an intense workout is a natural stimulant for the brain; better than any other. It engages the brain and brings it to a place of readiness. Physical activity brings forth changes in the brain that promotes the binding of brain cells. This is a process that is required for the brain to learn. Neil Duncan described the students as having heightened awareness. When asked to compare their current school experience to the previous year (prior to the experiment); the students mentioned feeling 'more awake' during school hours. Due to the undeniable success of this experiment, the school administration incorporated it into the high school curriculum and labelled it 'learning readiness P.E'.

To take it a bit further, the teachers decided to monitor 2 groups of literacy students. Both groups participated in the intense workout before school, but one of the groups had their literacy class straight after, whereas the other group waited until after the 8th period. Not a surprise to many that the group of students that had their literacy class straight after learning readiness P.E, performed better – achieving better literacy results than the group that had their class in the 8th period. Eventually this experiment spread throughout Naperville district, and the 19,000 students of this district became the fittest in the nation. The teachers provided a range of activities as an option, but the idea was to teach fitness and not sports. This created a health-aware lifestyle for them. The students in Naperville district didn't only become the fittest in the nation, they also became some of the smartest. Educators claim that spending a specific amount of money on pupils is a clear predictor of success. Naperville district spends below this amount – less than other top public schools in Illinois – but they consistently rank in the top 10 for academic performance in the state.

Studies show that children who exercise regularly, do the same when they are adults; reaffirming the initial beliefs of junior high teacher, Phil Lawler.

It's all in your head!

We could say the brain is a physical agent of the mind; in charge of our material functions. When your mind activates, your brain responds accordingly. Then your brain proceeds to give orders to the rest of the body. The information we allow our brains to receive, and then to signal; is of great importance. If the strength of the relationship between mind and matter isn't already evident, we can explore the effects that positive and negative thinking has on us – physically. Our brain is made up of two types of matter: white (60%), and grey (40%). Studies show that **positive thinking** increases grey matter in the pre-frontal cortex and in the hippocampus, benefitting memory and decision making. On the other hand, **negative thinking** not only causes a decrease in grey matter in the hippocampus; it also increases activity in the amygdala – responsible for activating the fight-or-flight response in the presence of a perceived threat.

In theory, it's easy to say we should just think positively all the time. In reality, that is difficult to do. Not because we lack the will, but because we may not be aware of our thoughts and where they came from. **Heterosuggestion** is the idea that outside sources may influence our subconscious thoughts, thus influence our behaviour. This can be from our parents, teachers, cultural norms, or even from our peers. These influences are most effective in our earliest years. Children are often referred to as sponges, for the way we absorb information in our environment at a young age. Beyond influencing what we deem as norms; these influences can tap into our emotions, and model how we behave in particular situations. **Autosuggestion** is the idea that we have the power to control our individual mind states. It can be conscious or unconscious, because it is based on what we tell ourselves. Where it gets tricky is that our autosuggestion could stem from prior heterosuggestion. Which is why we must be deliberate with our thinking, be positive in our thinking, and shape our behaviour accordingly. When in doubt, exercise!

Ways that exercise may positively navigate autosuggestion:

- Neuroplasticity – this is the brains ability to change itself by re-organising its structure and connections. When we exercise, brain plasticity is boosted. This allows mental adaptability, making it easier to form new habits.
- Feel-good hormones – when we exercise, several hormones are released which help improve our mood. When we are in a good mood, autosuggestion is more likely to be of a positive nature.
- Decrease in stress hormone – exercise suppresses cortisol, leaving us calm and mentally at peace.

According to the CDC (centers for disease control and prevention – US), your genes, your environment, and your habits are big factors in your overall health. What I find fascinating is that your behaviour and environment can cause alterations which influence the way your genes work. This is what is known as epigenetic changes. "Unlike genetic changes, epigenetic changes are reversible and do not change your DNA sequence. But they can change how your body reads a DNA sequence." - CDC. The National Center for Biotechnology Information states: "Research shows that the effects of trauma can be intergenerationally passed on through epigenetic mechanisms." Yikes! Studies have shown childhood trauma to cause epigenetic changes in human sperm. And these changes could be passed on generationally. Rachel Yehuda is a researcher who carried out intensive study on mass trauma survivors and their offspring. She concluded that trauma can be biologically passed down to the next generation, in order to "biologically prepare offspring for an environment similar to that of the parent." A recent study supported this belief, due to finding that children of holocaust survivors had different cortisol profiles to that of their peers; increasing the likelihood of anxiety disorders and PTSD. Don't worry, it's not all doom and gloom! Epigenetic changes could also be a good thing. Yes, stress can alter the behaviour of genes passed down by parents; but so can diet and exercise. According to studies, physical training can improve problem solving and memory, compared with those that do not partake in notable physical activity. Studies further show that the offspring of these active subjects will outperform the offspring of the sedentary subjects in a similar way. Exercising your body can make your kids smarter! Considering exercise is shown to suppress the stress hormone cortisol – increased by mental trauma – exercise will reduce the chances of that trauma causing epigenetic changes. This could potentially prevent these changes being passed on to offspring.

For all the negative impacts that heterosuggestion, autosuggestion, and trauma can have on the mind – which can influence us physically – exercise has numerous physical benefits that have a positive impact on the mind.

Mend with Movement

In psychology, trauma is described as an individual's experience of emotional distress from an event that overwhelms their capacity to respond to it.

Trauma is not only stored in the brain. This is according to Dr. Bessel van der Kolk, author of 'The Body Keeps the Score'. Trauma is stored in the nervous system and often bypasses the verbal memory pathways to then be encoded in the deep, non-verbal parts of the brain. This is a part of the brain that traditional talk therapy doesn't often reach alone. Movement-based practices, however, help to process and release trauma by engaging the body.

Trauma can disrupt communication between the prefrontal cortex – the rational, decision-making center – and the brainstem, which governs functions like heart rate, breathing, and the fight-or-flight response. What movement does, is help to reintegrate those systems. This allows the traumatised individual to regain emotional regulation and body awareness.

Due to its calming effects, some physical activity can activate the vagal nerve – reversing the constant state of fight-or-flight that is often caused by trauma. Movement becomes a form of expression that can release emotional experiences without the need for words.

High-intensity activities like sprinting or boxing can help discharge intense emotional energy. The traumatised brain craves structure and predictability. Rhythm-based activities like yoga or martial arts can provide this.

Help the body, help the mind!

This section is not to discredit the impact of traditional talk therapy, nor is it to suggest that one size shoe fits all. It is simply to highlight the healing potential of physical activity in relation to trauma.

"Traumatised people chronically feel unsafe inside their bodies: The past is alive in the form of visceral reactions..."

—Dr. Bessel van der Kolk

Get up, stand up – or rather, sit-up!

In a study carried out by the CDC (featured in the peer-reviewed medical journal The Lancet Psychiatry), results suggested that on average, a person has 3.4 poor mental health days per month. Poor mental health being, in this particular study; stress, depression, and emotional concerns. No surprise where I'm going with this one. Yes, you guessed it! The number of poor mental health days saw a reduction of nearly 50% amongst individuals that exercise. I could spend this whole chapter simply listing studies that support the same claims, but I'm sure by now you get the drift.

These benefits can be experienced through moderate, but regular exercise after just six months. The fluid IQ of the average person starts to decline during our 20s. However, many studies show that physical exercise is currently the only thing known that prevents this decline. A minimum of 150 minutes of exercise per week is what's recommended. A great place to start!

Can I have your attention!

It is widely accepted by experts that exercise can help individuals to manage their ADHD. Up to an hour of exercise 4 times a week can make a significant difference in ADHD symptoms.

Some of the reasons for this are as follows:

- Boosts dopamine, serotonin, and norepinephrine - people with ADHD are deficient in these neurotransmitters, which are crucial for improving attention and focus.
- Enhances memory and planning - commonly impaired in those with ADHD.
- Decreases hyperactivity - physical activity helps to channel excess energy in ways that are more productive. This can lead to a reduction in impulsive behaviours.

Routine and structure - organisation and predictability are known to help people with ADHD flourish.

Some of the best exercises for ADHD are aerobic activities such as running, cycling, and swimming. Team sports such as football and basketball are also hugely beneficial. Whilst disciplines such as boxing, martial arts, and even yoga, help to provide routine and structure while providing a physical outlet.

Get with the times!

This may be cliche, but it remains true that staying active can be fun. We constantly hear those from older generations – rightly or wrongly – speak on the issues that come with applications such as TikTok. My stance is that it is here now; so, let's think of how we can benefit from it instead of trying to avoid it completely. A common trend on TikTok is dancing of some sort. Dancing involves movement; physical exertion. I'm not savvy with social media, nor am I a great dancer (according to others), and I too used to reject these TikTok trends. But one day I saw the light. A friend told me to "stop being a grumpy old s*** and get with the times." And that I did. I began to understand the potential benefits – health related – that these platforms could offer.

CHAPTER 4

The best you!

The best you is a powerful you – physically and mentally. The relationship between physical power and mental power has been acknowledged in many cultures and philosophies.

Arete is a concept of ancient Greek culture that refers to excellence, purpose, fulfilment, or virtue. The center of this belief is about living up to one's full potential. In the eyes of the ancient Greeks – notably, philosophers such as Aristotle and Plato – excellence in mind, was developed through physical training. The gym was more than just a place for physical exercise; it was also for moral, and intellectual development. The Olympic Games was a clear reflection of this belief system. In the eyes of the ancient Greeks, athleticism was a symbol of human potential and internal greatness.

When building physical power, the body must face resistance. The foundation of power building is strength training. Power is rooted in strength; because your muscles will not be able to produce explosive force if they are not first strong. Strength training involves compound movements such as squats, deadlifts, bench presses, and overhead presses. These exercises develop overall strength. The idea is to lift heavy – it is recommended to train with 80-90% of your one-rep max (1RM) for low reps (3-6 reps per set). Gradually, you must increase the resistance, or the weight, to force adaptability and build strength. This is known as progressive overload.

After establishing strength, it is then necessary to incorporate plyometric training. This involves exercises such as box jumps, medicine ball throws, and clap push-ups. The reason for introducing plyometrics into the process is because these exercises train the muscles to produce force quickly. And this is what improves explosive power. The stronger you are, the more force you will produce. When strength training, it is recommended that we rest for 2-3 minutes between sets. For plyometric exercises, the recommended rest time between sets is 1-2 minutes.

Power is the result of force multiplied by velocity. Velocity represents the speed of movement. This means that once we establish force, it is important that we develop speed. When we train for speed, we improve movement efficiency and reaction times. Ladder drills, cone drills, sprints over short distances (10-40 meters), resisted sprints (up-hill, or with a sled), are some of the ways to improve speed.

The process of developing strength, then force, followed by speed, is what contributes to improved physical power. But to transfer that power effectively, you must develop your core. When speaking about the core, it is in reference to the group of muscles in your midsection that stabalise your spine and pelvis. This includes muscles in your back and your diaphragm, along with the abdominal muscles. The core acts as the primary stabaliser for your body. Therefore, the stronger it is, the more efficient your body will be. Some of the easiest ways to develop your core strength is by doing medicine ball twists, a plank, and hanging leg raises.

Though staying consistent is key; it is extremely important to avoid burnout. We must manage the workload by knowing how, and when to rest. Ideally, we should train power 2-3 times per week. If the muscles do not get adequate rest, they will not properly repair, nor grow.

Mentality

Improving the power of the mind is a similar process to that of physical power building. Strength is born out of resistance. In the case of the mind; resistance is adversity – a difficult or unpleasant situation. If the mind experiences – and overcomes – a difficult situation; growth will follow. Adversity is a privilege; it is needed for us to grow stronger. When this view is accepted, the voluntary adverse experience will feel less of a burden. Instead, it will be viewed as a necessity. As with building physical power, mental adversity can too be overwhelming. It is important to avoid mental burnout; therefore, having a mental break is necessary. Downtime varies depending on the individual, but the main idea is to have brief mental escapes from what predominately occupies your mind. What we must come to terms with; is the fact that power – whether physical or mental – cannot exist without discomfort. The world is a tough place; and in life, the strongest thrive.

Such thoughts are not alien to humanity. These views have been echoed across many regions throughout history. Ancient Indian warriors – notably those in the Kshatriya Caste, combined combat training and yoga. They believed that true mental power came as a result of training the body. Bushido: A Japanese philosophy which means "way of the warrior", is a moral code that was followed by the Samurai. This code of honour combines physical skill with mental and moral discipline. Mastery of martial arts was seen as a means to cultivate wisdom. For the Samurai, strength was about the overall mastery of oneself. Young Maasai warriors in Kenya undergo a rite of passage that contains intense endurance challenges. These challenges are seen as proof of both physical and mental power. Traditions such as these highlight the reality that physical and mental power are interconnected.

Resilience and approach – turning up the difficulty!

Physical fitness can be measured by monitoring improved strength, speed, or endurance. It is quantifiable. With character however, we can measure this through other means; such as resilience and discipline.

Resilience isn't built in comfort; it is forged in struggle. One way to measure resilience is by observing how you approach difficult tasks. For me, that task was hill sprints – particularly on cold mornings. I never looked forward to them, and I still don't. But over time, I noticed a shift. Initially, I'd delay getting out of bed. Once there, I'd even stretch longer than necessary, to delay starting. Now, I get up immediately and tackle the sprints head-on. The discomfort hasn't changed; my approach has. I still find the sprints difficult. They still hurt, and I still don't look forward to doing it. But I relish the challenge.

When the difficult task is a constant, a varying approach is evidence of increased, or reduced resilience. I took myself from a position of mental chaos to mental comfort – without changing the physical conditions. This change taught me that building resilience doesn't require drastic measures – just consistent effort. By confronting something challenging, like hill sprints, you train yourself to handle difficulty in other areas of life, whether it's a daunting work project or an overwhelming personal challenge.

This improvement for me wasn't deliberate. I was doing the hill sprints strictly for physical benefits. But after observing the other effects, I realised that we could tailor exercise routines to focus on the character-building aspect.

Our deepest responsibility

Life is tough, tricky, and often lonely. At times we feel stuck. This feeling often points to one root cause: a lack of purpose. Purpose is the fuel that drives motivation, and without it, we risk falling into stagnation – or even depression. Even on a fitness journey, we can feel stuck. That's when it's essential to recognise how fitness ties into life's overarching rules. Life – and fitness – is built on sacrifice. Growth requires us to let go of what we once valued, to attain something greater. We sacrifice late nights for productive mornings, indulgent meals for body goals, personal freedom for the needs of our children.

Sacrifice teaches us responsibility, and responsibility gives life purpose. Whether that responsibility is to others or simply to us, it creates a sense of direction and fulfilment. And when we take responsibility for becoming the best version of ourselves, we naturally fulfil our responsibilities to others.

Fitness is a microcosm of life. It's about sacrifice, progress, and purpose. Setting physical goals and pushing past your comfort zone awakens skills far beyond the physical. You gain discipline, broaden your perspective, and build resilience. These qualities help you not only reach your fitness goals but also grow into your best self.

Here's the truth: life is just a small part of what we call death. How we live now determines how we live forever – through the legacy we leave behind. Living intentionally, both in fitness and in life, ensures that our essence remains long after we're gone.

Let this mantra serve as a reminder and guide you: "My essence is here to stay. How I live forever is based on the effort I give today."

She changed up!

It had been a while since I'd spoken with a dear friend of mine. She moved away a few years ago to join the US air force; a dream she had for a little while. As she randomly crossed my mind, I decided to reach out to her. Upon answering the video call, it was hard not to notice her Saturn-like glow and gleeful smile. But I wasn't sure if that was down to her excitement in seeing me, or if it reflected how life had been treating her. Either way, I was happy. After some laughs and small talk, I said; "Paola, don't you have any regrets? Don't you miss your past life back here? You were doing well with work, and I'm quite sure you had an easier time." After an imperceptible laugh, she stated she will never regret becoming a better person. "The challenges I first faced in bootcamp, I can literally see how it's contributed to me having an easier time tackling other challenges in my life. The adversity I faced was to the point I didn't know how I would make it through the designated tasks. But I managed to. So for me to remember how I felt during those times, knowing that I still persevered, that was enough fuel to drive me through other struggles." I paused in awe; I found it admirable. But I was confused, because the Paola I knew was no stranger to exercise prior to joining the Airforce. The gym walls knew her face like she was an employee. My ignorance forced me to ask Paola how she feels the Airforce impacted her, differently to how her usual workout routines used to. She replied: "It unconsciously trained me to deal with uncertainty. Controlling my nerves, confronting things you can't prepare for. I'm the type of person who likes to have things under control, so I can prepare. But with the Airforce that wasn't possible. I had to deal with whatever life threw at me in that exact moment." Once again in awe; I was not only dumbfounded, but I was also inspired. At that very moment, I recalled what my uncle used to tell me as a child. "When exercising; you can push yourself to the point of discomfort. You can make yourself uncomfortable, very uncomfortable. But you will still be within your comfort zone."

It all clicked. What Paola was saying all made sense. And that's not to say you can't develop any self-improving skills/character traits through exercising by yourself, because you most certainly can (and we will explore that more). But traits such as dealing with uncertainty, is exclusive to having someone else pushing you.

She went on to tell me that her first reaction to most challenges was to make an excuse. This is an ugly habit to develop. I'm just glad, for her sake that the Airforce managed to break that habit. Being in the Airforce has taught her that her reasons (excuses) are just that; excuses! If old habits resurface and an excuse presents itself in response to a challenge, she quickly recognises that it's just nonsense. "I used to tell myself when I was in my hometown that I couldn't (didn't want to) do the push-ups that I was supposed to do if I didn't have a mat. But in bootcamp (in the Airforce) we were doing push-ups on our knuckles, on surfaces so hard it would make our hands bleed. This taught me many things, and one of those things was that every time I try to make an excuse, there is also a reason why it could be 10 times harder." Paola was always a straight talker, just like myself – which is probably why we always had transparency between us. She was as comfortable opening up to me as I was with her.

It brought me sincere joy hearing her speak about how focused she had become and how much she felt she had improved as a person. It was ironic how her mental strength and resilience had helped her develop her physical strength and resilience; which ultimately led to her being mentally strong and resilient - character! Mind boggling, I know. It's the whole chicken and egg argument; I don't know which came first, but what I do know is they go hand in hand.

Understandably enthralled by the conversation, I didn't take the time difference into consideration. My day was over, so I was relaxing. But Paola still had things to do. She mentioned an event she had to soon get ready for. I was shocked because if you know Paola, you would have known it takes her at least two hours to get ready for anything! So considering the time it was, and the time she had be at the event, I asked her why she was still wasting time on the phone to me instead of getting ready. Sarcastically, she asked if I had not been listening to anything she said in this conversation. "I am a changed woman!" I laughed and asked her what could the Airforce have possibly taught her about doing her make-up faster. She laughed and said, "if only that's what the Airforce was about, teaching us how to do make-up. We would lose every war." We both laughed. She followed up by saying, "To answer your question: A lot of routine. It gave me a lot of routine that I wasn't used to. It taught me the importance of being disciplined with timing and I was able to put that into practice when I began working." Me: "Explain, in what sense did it help you with that?" Paola: "TEN MINUTES! I learned the value of ten minutes. We had to get so much done; shower, clean up the area, all in ten minutes. This definitely made me more efficient in my overall life." The conversation ended not long after. We laughed, joked, and vowed to make a habit of having regular catch-up conversations. If each conversation is as enlightening as the first, I'll become wise in no time.

The things I learned from this conversation with my dear friend taught me a lot about the important role your mind plays in exercise. And in turn, the important role exercise can play in shaping your life for the better.

Don't underestimate the value of structure!

Time is the master; but master time

I often hear echoes of resistive diction when it concerns the dismantling of a comfort zone. As humans it is in our nature to resist any type of change, even if that change would benefit us. We like to feel as though there is nothing wrong with our current actions and we are in complete control of our circumstances. "My deeds are righteous, my actions are harmless, my lifestyle is not a concern." Deep down we all know the truth, whatever that may be. We bury reality because it is easier than accepting reality. No condemnation – naturally, we are all prone to this. This is the reason why regular introspection and self-reflection are necessary. What are we resisting, and will this resistance hinder our progress in any way? What can we implement to improve the structure of our lives? For years now I have taken the approach where the blame is always on myself. Even if on the surface I could point to reasons for a particular failure, or a not so gracious scenario; I will always dig deeper to figure out where it is I went wrong. There was something I did or did not do somewhere down the line that allowed this to happen. It is difficult to control the actions of others; but if I can identify, and then control my own actions, I will go a long way in my attempts to prevent the actions of others from influencing my outcomes. During my time working at the Holiday Inn hotel, there were many times where I was late to work, "through no fault of my own." My lateness led to a chain reaction.

Arriving to work late meant a colleague had to cover for me until my arrival. Meaning their day was interrupted in some way. This made me feel guilty. To compensate, I used to stay later after my shift. Staying later meant I was getting home later, leaving me with less time to cook. This resulted in me consuming a lot of fast food during that period.

I could continue to provide examples, but by now I believe I have painted a big enough picture to show how my lateness was impacting my days – as well as the days and the lives of others. But it was never my fault. The days I would drive to work, there was either an accident or another type of calamity. The drivers in front of me moving ridiculously slowly, or the number of temporary traffic lights along my route causing disruption to my journey. The days I would take the train to work; the service was poor, or the driver was moving too slow (I believe). After realising the impact that the constant lateness was having on my life, I decided to analyse it on a deeper level.

It did not make a difference whether I drove or used the train; my outcome was the same, and the only constant in that case, was me. What could I do to improve my circumstances? My commute to work was one hour, and after waking up in the morning, it would take me 45 minutes to get ready before I left for work. If I started at 9am, I would leave at 8am and wake up at 7:15am.

My first mistake was planning to get to work for the time I was due to start. If I aimed to get to work for 8:45am, I not only wouldn't have to move in a haste on arrival, but I would also be allowing for a 15-minute grace period in case there are any disruptions on my commute. If there are no disruptions, even better. I arrive to work early, settle in, and adequately prepare for the shift ahead. In theory, this sounded fantastic. If I were to just wake up fifteen minutes earlier, I could leave home fifteen minutes earlier, thus arrive to work in good timing.

But did I want to wake up fifteen minutes earlier? No. Why? That would mean I would be waking up tired due to having less sleep. Waking up tired could be the result of multiple factors (see section on sleep). But it's not by default I would get less sleep just because I'm waking up earlier. Surely, I could just go to sleep earlier the night before. This was the truth I did not want to acknowledge; it was too difficult. A lot of the time, trying to accomplish the greater good for something requires a lot of discipline. Discipline requires sacrifice. Sacrifice entails friction – something us humans naturally oppose. Another option to help me leave 15 minutes earlier would be to find a way to shorten the 45 minutes it takes me to get ready. How could I do this? Was I actually willing to spend less time in the shower? Either way I tried to look, the only doors in front of me to open involved a degree of sacrifice. That is when I realised that sacrifice is the essence of time management.

Time management is the ability to use one's time effectively or productively. It is the process of being punctual and/or carrying out set tasks in a manner which is efficient and non-disruptive to more of one's set tasks, or to the set tasks of others. In reality, how you manage your time could have a lot to do with your priorities. The level of importance you place on something may impact the urgency by which you approach it. When travelling abroad, I have no choice but to be meticulous when organising the day of my flight. I place a heavier importance on time management because of what is at stake. The domino effect to be had because of something as simple as waking up late on the day of a flight could lead to rushing when packing last minute items, leading to forgetting something – or even worse, missing the flight.

We must acknowledge the fact that the more important we regard a task, the more urgency we approach it with. However, it can be argued that our urgency is somewhat irrelevant. We can be aware of, and want to approach something in a particular manner, but not have the skills to do so. To briefly revisit the conversation I had with my friend Paola; initially she lacked the ability to be organised, despite knowing the potential implications of not being. It wasn't until she went through the bootcamp before she was able to be more efficient with her time – "ten minutes!" Yes, she had done this out of necessity, but also through deliberate practice. This is something every 'body' is capable of (see section on habit). Having good time management skills is advantageous because you are less of an inconvenience to others, meaning you could be favoured more in several instances. You are taken more seriously, known as someone that is able to stick to their word and follow through. This sense of reliability creates favour from employers and managers which could lead to making progressive steps in one's career. Lastly, if nothing else; through the development of time management skills, as an individual, you become more organised – making your life flow smoother. Just as poor time management produces negative domino effects, good time management does the opposite.

How do we improve our time management? One good aspect for good time management is having the ability to set micro targets within the overall target. To use getting to work on time as an example; I mentioned previously that I could attempt to shorten the time it takes me to get ready, to make this a possibility. Upon waking up, I would spend around 10 minutes in bed before getting up. My first adjustment would be to cut that 10 minutes down to 5. Next, instead of spending another 5 minutes arranging my belongings; I could do this the day before, as soon as I return home from work. Another 5 minutes saved. It is also not a necessity to stay longer in the shower just because I am enjoying the feeling of the water. Before I know it, I've cut 15 minutes off my routine without needing to lose any sleep. This of course, is just one example of how one could be more efficient with time. There is always a way to do so, even if it means sleeping earlier the night before so you could wake up earlier on the day of.

I must draw attention to the process of elimination used in the previous example. Being able to recognise the level of importance of each task or action is hugely advantageous for effectively managing time. By acknowledging the importance, or lack of, it will allow you to prioritise with wisdom. Therefore, you will waste less time on actions that have a lesser impact on your day. It is important to be realistic with your estimations. Can you realistically complete this task within 20 minutes, or is that estimation nothing more than hopeful? Be certain that the tasks you categorised as being less important, will not have a significant impact on your day. I cannot shower within 1 minute; nor can I get out of bed immediately after waking. Therefore, those are not things I would include in my time management plan. There is nothing more vital than being able to stick to your commitments.

My final point on this topic should provide more clarity regarding my first point. Relating to time management, it is necessary to acknowledge how important it is. Meaning when it has been done correctly or incorrectly, how it could bring forth negative or positive implications. This book is based on how physical activity is beneficial to the individual, the couple, and the group. The resistive diction regularly echoed as a reason for a lack of physical activity, is that of a lack of time. We should acknowledge just how high up on our list of priorities physical activity should be. With our furthered knowledge on how to better manage our time, we should be writing a plan centered around fitting any form of exercise into our schedules.

The 5-minute fix

Nobody is so busy that they don't have even 5-minutes in their day to dedicate to their health. For the busiest of individuals, here is a quick routine that you can incorporate in your day.

- 5 exercises
- 45 seconds work/15 seconds rest
- No equipment
- Can be repeated if you have more time

1. **Bodyweight Squats (45 sec)**
   Purpose: Legs, glutes, core
   If you need to modify: do half squats or sit to a chair and stand.
   Rest: 15 sec

2. **Push-Ups (45 sec)**
   Purpose: Chest, arms, shoulders, core
   If you need to modify: drop your knees or do wall push-ups.
   Rest: 15 sec

3. **Glute Bridges (45 sec)**
   Purpose: Glutes, hamstrings, low back
   Rest: 15 sec

4. **Plank Hold (45 sec)**
   Purpose: Core, shoulders
   If you need to modify: drop your knees or elevate hands on a surface.
   Rest: 15 sec

5. **High Knees (45 sec)**
   Purpose: Cardio boost, full-body activation
   If you need to modify: march in place for a low-impact version.

   Done!

Show up anyway!

CHAPTER 5

Every 'body' is different

Understanding always precedes conquer. In war, we must understand the weakness of our enemy, so we know what to exploit. In sport, we must understand how our opponent plays so we know how to restrict them. Even in seduction, we must understand our target, so we know how to attract them to us.

> *"If you know the enemy and know yourself, you need not fear the result of a hundred battles. If you know yourself but not the enemy, for every victory gained you will also suffer defeat. If you know neither the enemy nor yourself, you will succumb in every battle."*
>
> *- Sun Tzu, 'The Art of War'.*

But suppose the enemy of yourself, is yourself? And not in a mental sense. In this case, the "enemy" being your current physical state. Recognising the mental benefits that physical change can bring, and making the decision to implement the best changes for ourselves is a great starting place. But where do we go from there? Hitting the road and driving aimlessly is nice, and some argue that it's the better option. When we coast; we get a chance to clear our head and enjoy being present, without the stress of beating the clock. This can be beneficial, and at times necessary.

Another view is, when we have a destination and a map for the journey, our driving is more efficient. It's easier to keep going when we know we have somewhere to be. A clear destination, a route to get us there, and hopefully a car full of likeminded people. But how do we know where we want to go? And how do we get there? Understanding who we currently are (physically), is a must before mapping our journey.

A common method used to categorise our body composition, is the body type theory – somatotypes. This was proposed in the 1940's by William H Sheldon, PhD, M.D. According to the somatotype theory; our bodies can be analysed based on structure and thus placed into one (or more) of three groups. Those groups being: endomorph, mesomorph, ectomorph. These 3 body types are based on how the body stores and distributes fat. We will now explore each group in a little more detail.

Endomorph: These types tend to have a softer, rounder physique; with a wider frame, wider shoulders, wider hips and wider waist. As well as having a heavier bone structure, endomorphs have a higher composition of body fat, along with a slow metabolism; making it more difficult to burn calories.

Ectomorph: The ectomorph is naturally lean, and therefore has a narrow frame – shoulders, waist and hips. They find it easier to burn calories due to their fast metabolism and may find it challenging to gain muscle as a result.

Mesomorph: Naturally athletic with long limbs, broad shoulders and a narrow waist; the mesomorph gains strength easily. This type has a proportionate physique with defined muscle and has an easier time maintaining that muscle mass compared to other body types.

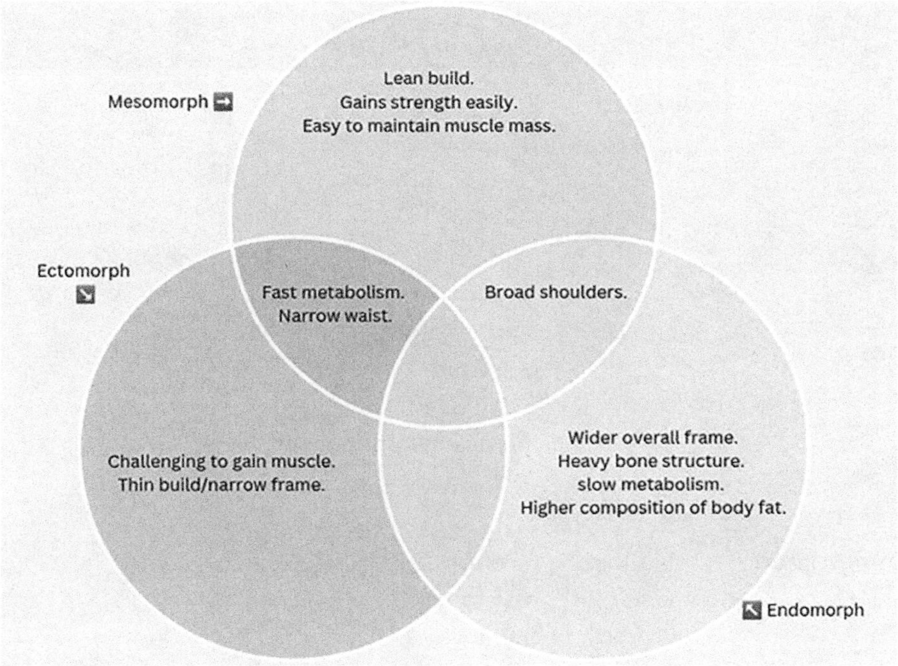

We may have preconceived ideas as to what a "fit" person looks like. But not looking a particular way does not mean that individual lacks fitness. There are more layers to it. Fitness is about being in the required condition for a specific task. For example, we may see an endomorph and assume they lack fitness. But that endomorph may be a shotput champion. They are fit for what their field requires but may not be fit to run a 10,000-meter race. Similar to how a long-distance runner may not be fit enough to successfully compete at shotput. Our body type can give us a natural advantage in a specific field over others who do not have the same somatotype. But regardless of our natural make-up, we can train our body for any purpose. We all have a unique vehicle; therefore, our journeys will be different. But the destination is always reachable.

The table below gives examples of some of the ways we can achieve specific results depending on our somatotype.

Somatotype	Target	Physical Activity	Diet
Ectomorph	Build muscle	Resistance training Compound exercises Strength training & progressive overload – gradually increase weight or intensity	Balanced mix of: Proteins – chicken, fish, tofu, legumes. Carbohydrates – wholegrains, sweet potato, fruits. Healthy fat – avocado, nuts, olive oil
Mesomorph	Maintain muscle	Strength & resistance training Body-weight exercises	Lean protein
	Gain healthy weight	Heavy weightlifting	Increase calorie intake with nutrient-dense foods – healthy fats, complex carbohydrates
	Lose muscle mass	Cardio – running, swimming, cycling	Reduce portion sizes. Choose different options – less calories

Endomorph	Build muscle	Strength & cardio - HIIT workouts	High-fiber foods: vegetables, fruits, whole grains.
	Lose fat	Cardio - running, swimming, cycling	Healthy fats (in moderation). Slow-digesting, high-fiber carbohydrates: sweet potato, quinoa, brown rice Lean protein

This table is a general guideline. For a more personalised solution, it may be more impactful to seek consultation.

Refrain from shame; all bodies are not the same!

Personality in fitness

Every 'body' is different physically, but we also differ in who we are, beyond the physical. When we describe people beyond their physical features, we usually consider their personality. This way of categorising humans is very common.

Personality is a combination of how an individual thinks, feels, and behaves – on a consistent basis. How we feel may influence how we think; which in turn, may dictate how we behave. Our interests are an expression of all 3.

There is a popular personality test known as the Myers-Briggs Type Indicator (MBTI). This test was developed by Katherine Cook Briggs, and her daughter Isabel Briggs Myers. According to MBTI, there are 16 personality types by which individuals can be categorised. The concept of this test is based on psychiatrist Carl Jung's theory of "psychological types".

Jung's claim was that we can be categorised in 4 dichotomies, according to our preferences.

Those dichotomies:

- Extraversion (E) or Introversion (I)
- Sensing (S) or Intuition (N)
- Thinking (T) or Feeling (F)
- Judging (J) or Perceiving (P)

When each of these are combined, there are 16 potential outcomes (personality types). This is how the MBTI was birthed.

Here is a breakdown of the 16 different combinations:

1. INTJ – This type is a visionary. Strategic in how they approach tasks, they make planning for the future enjoyable.
2. INTP – This type thrives when having to understand complex systems. They are problem solvers. And due to their innovative and curious nature, they love exploring ideas and theories.
3. ENTJ – These types are bold, ambitious leaders who excel in the face of challenge. A strong trait of the ENTJ is their ability to organise people and resources. They are very decisive and goal oriented.
4. ENTP – They love to explore new possibilities. Their quick-wit helps them during debates – which is something they love. These types are very energetic.
5. INFJ – Despite being private and pragmatic, these types are very caring. Their aim is to make the world a better place. The INFJ is very insightful.
6. INFP – These types focus on self-expression and the understanding of others. Due to being deeply in tune with their values, they often express compassion. The INFP are deeply imaginative individuals.
7. ENFJ – Charismatic and inspiring leaders who enjoy motivating others. These types are empathetic; therefore, they excel in relationship building.

8. ENFP – Open-minded, creative, and enthusiastic. These types love to connect with others and explore new ideas.
9. ISTJ – These types place value on tradition. They excel in creating structure and efficiency. The ISTJ is organised and dependable.
10. ISFJ – They are detail-oriented. The ISFJ is caring. As a loyal protector, they express their care through their desire to help others.
11. ESTJ – Strong-willed, organised, natural leaders. Efficiently managing projects and people, is where the ESTJ best thrives.
12. ESFJ – They are attuned to the needs of others. Due to how much they value harmony, they are often the glue that holds the group together.
13. ISTP – Practical and hands-on problem-solvers. They love working with tools and exploring how things work.
14. ISFP – Artistic and free-spirited individuals who value self-expression and authenticity. These types are highly attuned to their surroundings.
15. ESFP – Spontaneous and social. They enjoy entertaining others, and they love new experiences.
16. ESTP – These types love to take risks, and they enjoy making things happen in the moment. They are bold, energetic, and action oriented.

Each of us will identify best with one of these 16 types. There are online tests that can provide an accurate indication for which suits you best. Knowing your personality type can be beneficial when determining which forms of physical activity will suit you best. Some people are forever turned away from exercise simply because the type of exercise they attempted wasn't enjoyable for them. One way to avoid this is by making your choices of exercise align with your personality. This creates a better chance of a longer-term commitment.

Below is a table detailing the physical activities that best align with each personality type.

Type	Physical Activities	Reason
INTJ	Martial Arts e.g. Jiu-jitsu, Taekwondo, boxing.	These activities offer strategic, disciplined practices that align with their desire for mastery.
INTP	Rock climbing, archery, fencing. Cycling, running, swimming.	The first 3 of these activities include problem-solving and concentration; which appeals to the analytical nature of the INTP. The solo activities allow them to have time to think deeply and self-reflect.
ENTJ	Competitive team sports e.g. basketball, football.	These sports align with their leadership qualities, and their desire for structured challenges.
ENTP	Dancing, team sports, fencing.	These activities either provide a fast-paced, unpredictable situation, a mental battle, or a fun expressive outlet.
INFJ	Yoga, Tai Chi.	These practices foster mindfulness, alignment with personal values, and a sense of inner peace.
INFP	Hiking, pilates.	Solitary, nature-focused activities allow for introspection and creativity.
ENFJ	Spin classes, zumba, team sports.	These activities align best with the ENFJ because they enjoy working with others in collaborative environments.
ENFP	Dance, surfing.	These are creative and adventurous activities that offer excitement and freedom of expression.

ISTJ	Golf, running.	Individual activities that are centered on a goal. These suit the disciplined and methodical approach of the ISTJ.
ISFJ	Swimming, cycling.	These activities provide a calming, health-focused environment that aligns with the caring and dependable nature of the ISFJ.
ESTJ	Tennis, rowing.	Competitive and structured sports appeal to their leadership and goal-setting tendencies.
ESFJ	Volleyball, dance classes.	These social, cooperative activities align with the ESFJ's love of teamwork and connection.
ISTP	Mountain biking, kickboxing.	The ISTP loves hands-on, fast-paced activities that require skill and precision.
ISFP	Stand-up paddleboarding, figure skating.	Artistic and outdoor sports, allows the ISFP to express themselves authentically.
ESTP	Football, snowboarding.	High-energy, fast-paced sports align with their need for thrill and action.
ESFP	Dance (salsa, hip-hop), cheerleading.	These lively activities allow them to shine, and to connect with others.

The above table is a guideline for those struggling to find a type of exercise that best fits them as an individual. This could be for oneself, or it could be a guide for a parent seeking the best activity/activities for their child(ren) to take part in.

Archetypes

Our individual attitude towards physical activity reflects our overall, deeper character. Based on my observations, I have come up with 4 archetypes that define our approach to exercise, and life overall.

The 4 archetypes:

1. The All or nothing Achiever
2. The Grinder
3. The perfectionist
4. The Tinkerer

The All or Nothing Achiever

Core traits:

- High expectations for themselves
- Intensity-driven
- Obsessed with momentum and performance
- Struggles with moderation
- Prone to burnout

Breakdown:

This type is never one foot in with anything. If they don't believe they can do a task to a high enough standard, they would rather not be involved at all. They either fully commit to something with tunnel vision, or they completely avoid it. The all or nothing achiever ties their value to exceptional performance. They find it discomforting if they are not the best. To them, being average feels like failure.

They avoid challenges that are unfamiliar; because avoiding the possibility of failure protects their self-image. Being in an unfamiliar situation may expose a weakness in their ability. On the flip side, the tasks they do participate in, they approach with intensity.

How this archetype approaches exercise:

- Starts new routines with maximum intensity
- May be driven by a big event (vacation, wedding)
- Not meeting expectations leads to completely boycotting the plan
- May swing back and forth between intense training phases and complete inactivity

Ways to improve their approach to exercise/life:

- Focus on consistency rather than intensity. 15-minutes is better than zero
- Become more immersed in the process instead of obsessing over the outcome
- Acknowledge progress rather than being driven by perfection
- Stop avoiding risk and start being curious about growth – effort is excellence

Practical exercise suggestions to help overcome the less glamorous habits:

- Try something new – forces openness and patience. E.g. taking up a new sport can teach them not to tie their value to exceptional performance, but to find value in effort and the willingness to improve.
- Create a habit based on a streak – They learn to value consistency and repetition over intensity. For example, do 10/15-minutes of light movement each day, despite how one is feeling. Walking, jogging, stretching are good activities for this. Consistency builds character.
- Group training – reduces the likelihood of being the best. Being in this situation disrupts the ego loop. team sports or combat sports gyms are ideal. When consistently exposed to an environment where they are not the best, it may encourage them to focus more on progression.

- Slow exercises – teaches patience and long-term focus. There is not always a need for intensity. Activities like yoga are perfect for this.
- High-intensity sprint session – feeds their need for intensity, but forces rest. When doing a high-intensity sprint session, maximum rest between sets is required. This is so that each sprint can be completed with maximum effort. 6-10 maximum effort sprints with a 5/6-minute rest between each can train the mind of the All-Or-Nothing achiever to see that high performance in any setting requires adequate rest periods. This approach will help them to avoid burnout across the board.

The All or Nothing Achiever has the potential to do great things. But to do that, they must first broaden their outlook.

The Grinder

Core traits:

- Resilient
- Disciplined
- Hardly makes excuses
- Emotionally steady
- Rigid

Breakdown:

The Grinder is the type that sticks to a plan regardless of the circumstances. They keep the long-term goal in sight, pushing through discomfort and resisting the lure of instant gratification. Their discipline and work-ethic is evidence of their commitment. That commitment however, could be a double-edged sword. With The Grinder, signals of distress or exhaustion are often ignored. They view excuses as a sign of weakness. Their heightened focus makes them tunnel visioned. This leaves no room for flexibility in their strategy or routine.

How this archetype approaches exercise:

- Consistently shows up
- Does well with long-term programs
- Gives maximum effort
- May use exercise as an outlet for control
- Prone to burnout
- Rigid with routines

Ways to improve their approach to exercise/life:

- Introduce variety in routine – without compromising consistency
- Encourage enjoyable activities – not always hard, grueling exercises
- Reframe rest as a major contributor to the overall goal – recovery is required for growth
- Data tracking – monitor variability in heart rate – they get in the habit of knowing when to tone it down

Practical exercise suggestions to help overcome less glamorous habits:

- Yoga – slows them down and forces introspection
- Skill-based activities (Olympic lifting, martial arts) – shifts focus from just grit to coordination
- Strength training with de-load phases – highlights the important role of rest for overall growth

Once The Grinder understands who they are, implementing some of these routines will go a long way. The shift in mindset will make The Grinder more fluid in their approach to goals, by acknowledging the value of rest and recovery.

The Perfectionist

Core traits:

- Overthinker
- Attention to detail
- High standards
- Loyal to routines once confident
- Self-reflective
- Focused on growth

Breakdown:

The Perfectionist finds comfort in certainty. They are often well-researched, self-aware, and highly intelligent. Their need for doing things 'right' can sometimes be a hindrance to their progress. This is because they usually delay starting something because of the fear of doing it 'wrong'. To this archetype, if it's not perfect, it's not worth doing. Driven by improvement and long-term success, The Perfectionist does endless research and looks for the 'best' options. In relation to exercise, that would mean the 'best' routine, diet, and even gear.

How this archetype approaches exercise:

- Does endless research – watches tutorials, compares programs
- Extremely focused (at times, too much) on form and execution
- May end the session if something feels off
- May constantly compare themselves to others – often unfairly down-playing their own abilities

Ways to improve their approach to exercise/life:

- Appreciate progress over perfection
- Practice being sooner to act rather than over-planning
- Commit to working on weaknesses

Practical exercise suggestions to help overcome the less glamorous habits:

- Group classes (pilates, spin, HIIT) – this takes away the burden of figuring out the 'best' plan
- Boxing (boxercise) – this encourages gradual 'perfection'. Being vulnerable in unfamiliar territory is one thing, but doing that in a group setting introduces a different dynamic
- Dance classes – encourages The Perfectionist to follow through with the session despite the inevitable constant mistakes

The Perfectionist is an interesting archetype. The key to their character progression is to recognise the situations where they need, and do not need to be so diligent. Once that is mastered, this archetype can truly thrive in any field

The Tinkerer

Core traits:

- Loves trying new things
- Gets bored easily by routine
- Curious
- Creative
- Reflective
- At times can lack consistency

Breakdown:

If one doesn't understand The Tinkerer, they may view them as inconsistent. This is because they are more driven by refinement than they are by routine. Tinkerers adjust routines to better suit themselves. They often do this through trial and error; teaching themselves along the way. Their reflective nature makes them constantly analyse their progress. And to aid their progress – from their perspective – they may end a current routine for a completely new one.

How this archetype approaches exercise:

- Constantly switching it up – prone to trying new classes, new programs
- Starts enthusiastically, but may struggle to follow through
- Lover variety and avoids repetitive work
- Approach to tasks may be driven by emotion – their mood or energy levels can dictate their commitment
- They could create a new warm-up based on how their body feels that day
- May monitor data like heart rate or track their rest time just for fun

Ways to improve their approach to exercise/life:

- By understanding that not everything can or will be personalised to suit their feelings
- Incorporate variety into a consistent program
- Using different challenges to maintain engagement over longer time periods

Practical exercise suggestions to help overcome the less glamorous habits:

- Calisthenics and bodyweight training – plenty variety to avoid boredom
- Functional training (squats, lunges, plank) – encourages creativity in movement sequencing
- Olympic lifting – a skill-based exercise that appeals to their fondness of refinement

The Tinkerer has all the tools to become one of the most innovative, self-directed movers of all. But first, this problem-solving archetype must see the value in consistency. They must see boredom not as a cue to quit, but as a test of resolve. With this slight shift in mindset, the world is at their feet.

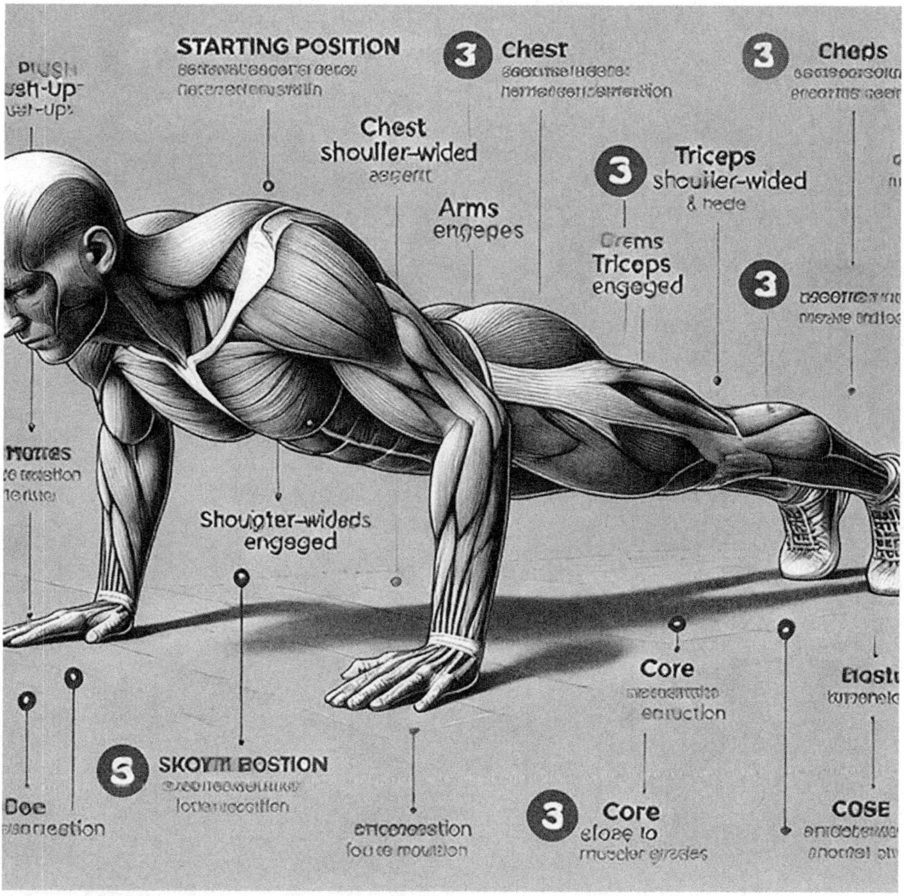
STARTING POSITION
3 Chest
3 Cheds
Chest
shouller-wided
3 Triceps
shouiler-wided
Arms
engepes
Tricops
engeged
3
Shougter-wideds
engeged
Core
3 Core
COSE

CHAPTER 6

Do for love

Self-Love is a state of appreciation for oneself that grows from actions that support our physical, psychological and spiritual growth. Self-love means having a high regard for your own well-being and happiness. Self-love means not settling for less than you deserve. - Jeffrey Borenstein, M.D.

A Fatal Realisation

Joseph Cartagena, a native to New York City, had many struggles growing up. He came from a financially challenged family in the poorer parts of The Bronx. However, deprivation and crime weren't the only struggles Joseph endured as a child. Unfortunately, at the age of just 14, he was diagnosed with diabetes. Despite street politics and legal troubles, Joseph managed to find success in the music industry, after being introduced to rap by his brother. Not only did he become a successful rapper himself, but he also founded his own label that he has successfully ran since its existence. His label has been home to many successful acts; notably his mentee and good friend, Christopher Rios.

Christopher Rios, also from The Bronx in New York City; was a high school drop-out. Despite that, he had an intelligent way with his words. He was the naturally athletic type, playing many sports growing up. Mainly basketball and boxing (this was despite breaking his leg at a young age). His perseverance and intelligent wordplay contributed to him becoming a successful rapper and finally escaping the shackles of poverty. But despite becoming a success in his field, it wasn't enough to rid his mind of his troubled childhood. After all, who wouldn't be troubled by witnessing heinous crimes at a young age, whilst being a victim of abandonment that led to homelessness at the age of 15. This trauma, added with the pressures of being a young father, caused Christopher to start over-eating – his way of coping. He found comfort and love in food, instead of finding it within himself (not that it was easy to do so). Within just 3 years; between the ages of 18 and 21, Christopher gained 120lbs (54 kilograms), bringing his weight to 300lbs at that time. Over-eating and drug abuse led to an alarmingly rapid rise in Christopher's weight. This caused his good friend and mentor, Joseph to intervene.

Joseph convinced Christopher to attend a diet program at The Duke University. This was beneficial because Christopher managed to lose 80lbs (35 kilograms) during that time. However, he quit the program before its completion, and he ended up gaining more weight. In one of his hit songs; titled "It's So Hard", Christopher said the line "I just lost a hundred pounds (lbs) I'm tryna live". Despite this alleged weight loss, he not long after suffered a heart attack – due to his obesity. As a result of the heart attack, he died. He was 29 years old at the time of his death, and he left behind a wife and three children. His wife said: "He was depressed, he really wasn't happy with himself." He weighed 700lbs (300 kilograms) at the time of his death.

Joseph Cartagena who was the mentor and friend of the late Christopher Rios, had also struggled with obesity. He said; "I went to his (Christopher's) funeral, and I felt like Ebenezer Scrooge. Like, I'd seen me. And I'm looking at his little daughter. I said to myself, you lose weight, otherwise you're outta here." The process was difficult for Joseph, who himself fell into depression after the death of his good friend. His depression lasted two years, during which time he had gained significant weight; ultimately reaching 470lbs (213 kilograms). He finally reached a point where he told himself enough is enough and started his weight loss journey. Joseph did everything he could to reach a healthier weight. He ran on treadmills; wearing sweatsuits, and he implemented strict diet plans. His efforts paid off because he managed to lose 200lbs (90 kilograms); and in doing so, he says he cured his depression.

For Joseph, this was more than a phase, it became a lifestyle. He continues to exercise; and regularly checks his blood pressure, cholesterol and blood sugar levels so that he can stay on top of his health. Thankfully, his latest health choices led to the eradication of his diabetes – which had plagued him since the age of 14. "I was a diabetic for 16 years, since I was 14. Being that I lost weight, no more diabetes. You don't have to lose your eyesight, cut off your toes, have a stroke, get kidney failure." After this realisation; it's no surprise why Joseph was able to not only shed the weight, but to keep it off.

"When you're fighting yourself there isn't a wall high enough that you can build. There isn't an island you can run to. There isn't a place you can go to where you can get away from it, because you're fighting your mind." - Joseph Cartagena, aka 'Fat Joe'.

A closer look

Some argue that self-love is immeasurable; and synonymously, a spectrum. They claim there are varying amounts of self-love, specific to the individual. I can offer another perspective, however. It can also be argued that self-love is black and white. You either have it or you don't, and how we measure that, is through action. It can be viewed as a verb, rather than an immeasurable claim. Otherwise, how would we know whether it exists?

Self-love is absolute, but the ways in which it is expressed is what varies. Love is the act of doing what we feel is best for the individual in each moment, which will have instant or long-term effects. It differs from admiration, obsession, and infatuation. We could simply admire someone without acting on the admiration. We could admire musicians, teachers, health officials and sportspeople; but are we willing to do what is best for them despite the sacrifice that could be required of us? I doubt that. When we speak about infatuation, we're speaking about something without rationality. It's a short-lived feeling that is difficult to justify. The feeling, and or behaviour is not linear to the relationship with the individual. Infatuation can be a rocket into the black hole of obsession, and that's where things get tricky. Obsession is a pre-occupation with something or someone, with the potential of it not only becoming a dominant force in your mind, but also in your life. Having an obsession towards something or someone isn't necessarily about doing what's best for that individual. Which is why, without love; obsession can be harmful. Obsession and love can co-exist. Think of love as a plate of food; indeed, I can eat with my hands, but a knife and fork can be more than useful in assisting my fullness. Therefore, if fullness is the goal, a knife and fork can be a useful tool to help me consume the food. Love is unconditional. It is sacrifice; it is compromise of our comfort. Love is about action through deep affection, despite these inconveniences. Therefore, self-love, would mean constantly showing up for us no matter how uncomfortable it makes us.

The fact that I love myself (even though there's been times where I haven't) makes me do what is best for my health, to the point where at times it had become an obsession (a healthy one). Due to my poor eating habits, at a particular time in my life my blood sugar level was higher than I would have liked. Because of this, I took it upon myself to act. I started being strict with my food consumption until I saw a change. And now; although there are still times I give in to my unhealthy cravings, it certainly isn't enough to cause me harm. I make a conscious effort with this. Just as I make an effort to run miles on a regular basis, despite my hatred for running. This is an example of how love can be expressed through discipline – similarly to how one can be faithful to their spouse. And my obsession with my health, is demonstrative of the love I have for myself.

I was once told by a teacher that you deserve everything you desire; if what you desire, you are willing to work for. We all desire more, it's human nature. But 'more' looks different for each of us. Some desire more money; others desire more friends. Regardless of what it is, everything can be reachable with a plan. Having an idea is the foundation, but a plan is an elevator to accomplishment. The will in which we attempt to execute a plan is tied to the level of want. Apply that sentence to the topic of self-love. A strong want of the best outcome for ourselves, will lead to us planning, and doing what will take us there. It ends with us, and it starts with us. Let's be happy with the realisation that we want what's best for ourselves. It's a positive realisation, regardless of whether we are already on, or are currently thinking about taking action. I know it's easier said than done, and I've been there myself. Approaching this with positivity is more effective. Loving yourself by seeking better for yourself, is somewhat of a craving for positivity. Acknowledge this. many of us are guilty of letting the world around us affect our thoughts and actions. When in actuality, real strength is letting our thoughts and actions affect the world around us. It sounds ludicrous, but we should be more childlike in some of the ways we approach life. There is beauty in it. As adults we look out of a window and see dirty puddles caused by rain, we see pollution, we see strangers that could be a danger to us. When a child looks out of a window, the child sees a rainbow caused by rain, they see fresh air, they see people they can make friends with. In a child's eyes; many things are possible, and they are. At times, we're all guilty of thinking the best outcomes could never be for us, but they can. That's not to say we will all win the lottery, no. That is out of our hands. But it is impossible to win the lottery if you refuse to buy a ticket. As for your well-being, the ticket is already in your possession. Being impatient at times is natural. Being discouraged during the journey is natural. But if the want for being better remains, you must keep showing up for yourself - putting action behind those thoughts.

CHAPTER 7

The Character of Habit

Cambridge Dictionary's description of habit: 'Something that you do often and regularly, sometimes without knowing that you are doing it'.

If there is one thing I've learned from boxing, it's that your habits always reach the surface. These behavioural patterns are so deeply ingrained in us. It's almost like our fingerprint. But what differentiates our habitual proclivities from a fingerprint, is that we can change them. We weren't born with our current habits; we developed them at different stages of our lives. The concept of habit, relating to humans, shows how primitive we are. But what separates us from other animals is the capacity that we have to create or manipulate our habits; and this gives us the ability to override the 'bad' ones. At times, we are slaves to our subconscious. But the same thing that makes us slaves, is the same thing that makes our lives easier.

Think of the times you've been on the way home and in need of the toilet. Why is it that the closer you get to your house, the need to use the toilet becomes greater? This can be interpreted as an unconscious message from the mind, telling the body to prepare to release urine – because your toilet is now within your reach. Have you ever wondered why the more time we spend lying in bed – regardless of the length of time we've been rested – the more sluggish or tired we feel. This could be because our mind associates our bed with sleep, therefore it sends a signal to our body, telling it to enter a state of relaxation.

What is known in psychology as the law of association, is based on the fact; that no idea exists in the mind except in association with other ideas... Memory is the primary representative faculty or power of the mind. - William Atkinson.

One Friday, on a rainy autumn evening, I arrived home after coaching 6 sessions. Not necessarily tired but certainly wanting to relax. I usually meal-prep enough food to last me from Sunday to Thursday; allowing for some flexibility on Fridays and Saturdays. Though I say flexibility, I'm usually rigid in my selection. As a child, after school on a Friday evening; we would order pizza and eat it together as a family, while watching a movie. I continued doing this during my adult years - it eased my mind, for whatever reason. This Friday in particular, as I waited for my tuna pineapple pizza; the movie I decided to watch was called "50 First Dates". The synopsis of this movie; is that a man (Henry), falls in love with a woman (Lucy), who unfortunately suffered a bad car accident a year prior to him meeting her - leaving her with short term memory loss. Every day she woke up, she believed it was the same date it was when her accident took place. Lucy's recollection of the previous day, the next day, was always non-existent. Therefore, any events after her accident, or anyone she met, was a futile experience. As a result, Henry, had numerous 'first dates' with Lucy - in what eventually became a successful attempt to win her over. Although this movie was just a comedy, and not based on any true story, I wondered how realistic it was for someone to develop a condition similar to the one portrayed by Drew Barrymore (Lucy).

After some research, I found many answers. I came across the case of Eugene Pauly – a historical case. Eugene Pauly suffered from Retrograde

Amnesia – similar to the Anterograde Amnesia suffered by Lucy in '50 First Dates'. The only difference is that Anterograde Amnesia prevents the formation of new memories; whereas, Retrograde Amnesia is the inability to remember experiences from the past, while also not being able to store new information.

This is why the Eugene Pauly case was groundbreaking; because it was through this case, scientist Larry Squire discovered the important role habit played in memory formation, thus behaviour. Eugene Pauly could recover memories from earlier on in his life, but the memories within roughly thirty years prior to his infection (that caused his amnesia), were absent. Due to his Retrograde Amnesia, Pauly would have to be accompanied by a family member whenever he left the house, otherwise there was a likelihood he wouldn't make it back. He would ask the same questions daily, receiving the same answers - to no future benefit, as he would eventually forget. He wouldn't remember the day of the week, nor even his own children. His wife would take him for daily walks. However, one day when she was upstairs getting dressed, she realised Eugene was gone. In a state of panic, she rushed outside to look for him, having no success. After 15 minutes or so, she went back inside to alert the local authorities, only to find Eugene sitting, watching television. He had no recollection of leaving the house, or even coming back in. But his wife knew he had left because of the state of his hands, along with some of the things on the table that he could have only collected from outside.

Pauly was able to find his own way home after a walk, despite having impaired memory. Because of this breakthrough, Squire carried out further experimental tests on Pauly, which guided him to the understanding of how habit works.

Our bodies get us to repeat behaviour that is in the best interest of our bodies - Simon Sinek.

Let's interpret "the best interest of our bodies" as simply, effort saving; whether good or bad for us. Due to the formation of habits, the brain has less work to do; less thinking – making it more efficient. The more our brain functions on autopilot, the more room it has for other problems. If most of our daily challenges are habitual, the brain is less overwhelmed, which means it requires less space. This leads to the head becoming smaller, making childbirth more efficient. This is one of the ways our brain creates habits for the best interest of our body. However, developing a habit for efficiency doesn't necessarily mean the habit is good for us. For example, the consumption of fast food can become a habit. Even though this is a conscious habit, it could be one that is hard to stop. Just as on the flip side, exercise such as running, can also become habitual. With that being said, not all of our habits – good or bad – are conscious.

Most of my observations were obtained through boxing. I would see trends while watching or participating and try to apply them to the outside world. In boxing, some fighters may have a (good) habit of bringing their hand back to their face after throwing a punch. Whereas others may have a (bad) habit of keeping their chin in the air. When conscious, most can implement certain (good) actions. However, in a moment where thinking time is limited, everyone will revert to what is habitual. The same applies in life. And something else that applies in boxing, that is also true in the real world, is that we can make the instant reaction into what we want it to be; through repetition.

The Basal Ganglia is the part of the brain which assists us in habit formation, and then programs us with those habits, making them automatic responses. When we are performing tasks, this part of the brain is the most actively engaged - even if the rest of the brain is not active at all. However, the more we repeat a task; the less active the Basal Ganglia, and the overall brain becomes. This is because when repeated consistently, a task becomes habitual, therefore less thinking is required. Maybe after a month (or less than, depending on the individual) of driving home from a new job, on a route that was once new to a person; one may, or may not notice that the levels of concentration required to get home has decreased. Less looking at road signs or maps, and more daydreaming, or even fully engaging in the music being played in the car. Before you know it, you are back home. Just as my five-year-old nephew was able to walk us to his house when I picked him up from school; despite not being able to explain the directions. This is how Pauly managed to find his way home after disappearing for a walk – through unconscious familiarity. His brain was able to recognise, and store repeated behaviour.

The formula behind habit formation is: cue-action-reward. The cue being the trigger; this is what brings about the response. For example, if I smelled something unpleasant, the unpleasant smell is the cue - triggering the response (action) of me covering my nose. The reward I get is I've stopped myself experiencing the unpleasant smell. Similarly, in boxing; the cue is a jab coming my way - the response is me blocking it with my right hand - the reward is me not getting hit. Keeping with boxing, a negative example would be; a punch coming towards me (cue) - automatic response (action/reaction) of me lifting my chin in the air - the reward (or punishment in this case) is me getting hit with the punch. Getting hit would not be in my best interest. Therefore, for my own good I would be forced to exercise discipline, by creating a habit that leads to a better reward. If one lacks the ability to apply discipline inside of the ring, they will lack that same ability outside of the ring - and vice versa.

In October 2020, a boxing match that gained worldwide viewership, took place. That match being; Davis vs Santa Cruz. In this fight, it was picked up by the commentary that Santa Cruz had a bad habit of dropping his right hand after throwing it. This was something he did continuously since the start of the fight. Whether Santa Cruz was conscious or unconscious of this action; it made no difference, because it was a habit, and a habit is not something that can be changed instantly. It was habitual because it is what he does when training, therefore when in the fight, his body is already programmed to do the same. Whenever Santa Cruz threw the punch and dropped his right arm, he left his chin exposed. His opponent, Davis, understanding the science behind habitual behaviour in boxing, noticed this habit and capitalised. He waited for Santa Cruz to throw his right hand again, knowing he will drop it afterwards. He (Davis) then threw a perfectly timed uppercut, which landed on the exposed chin of Santa Cruz. The fact of habit is why boxers, together with their coaches' study footage of their opponents prior to a fight. They analyse certain negative habitual traits of a fighter, in the hope of structuring a game plan that they can use to capitalise on it.

Danger, or the anticipation of danger, may send us into a fight or flight response. When in this fight or flight mode, our most instinctive behaviours surface. Knowing this, it would be prudent to program our body to respond positively when in such situations. An example; staying calm when under pressure - this is a transferable trait. One way to develop this positive response, is through boxing training. A boxing training environment provides a perfect blend of fear, courage, discipline and habit exposure. According to psychologists; when one deliberately exposes themselves to a phobia, they have a good chance to overcome it. Whereas when exposed to the same phobia unintentionally, that phobia becomes worse.

Be deliberate!

Arousing your taste buds, giving in to your cravings provides you with a dopamine hit. This dopamine hit is the reward of consuming sugary/salty/oily foods. The cue can range from a smell, a television commercial, a particular day of the week, or even simply finishing work. Having a heart attack due to this habit could be the long-term reward (punishment). The negative result of this habit could be the window to developing a habit with a more positive long-term reward. It has been observed that the best way to stick to a newly introduced exercise routine is by choosing a very specific and comprehensible reward. For example: a cue of getting out of bed every morning, an action of doing fifty press-ups because of the cue, and a reward of having an extra croissant with breakfast; because of the action. This reward is guilt-free because it is based on the idea that the extra croissant was earned - due to the action of doing press-ups. We train dogs in the same way. It is about creating habits; based on a cue (command) - a response (the action we reinforce) - a reward (pat on the head or a treat).

According to studies, just under 50% of the US population make resolutions at the turn of a new year. Many of these resolutions are health based: exercising more, eating better etc. However, it is said that nearly half of these people fail in their attempts. Experts say the reason for failure is the negligence of self-directed neuroplasticity - a term first defined by research psychiatrist, Jeffrey M. Schwartz. Self-directed neuroplasticity is the process of intentionally rewiring one's brain, to create positive habits.

Many of our resolutions and overall goals are difficult. They are usually targets for us to reach, so that we can be better versions of ourselves in some way. A lot of the time, what is good, does not come easy. Success of any kind requires some type of discipline and structure. The key is structuring that structure. It is best to start small. Break down long term destinations into different streets. Each street with their own junction, their own service station, but all leading to the same place. If we paid enough attention when looking around, we will notice routine and habit in most situations. Content creators have to follow a routine; just as the creators of the apps that those content creators use had to. Even the apps themselves function based on specific structures; and they sometimes have cues that lead to actions and outcomes.

It has been established that habits are our instinctive actions. If we agree that habits are transferrable – how we do one thing is how we do everything. Therefore, a collection of our habits, is essentially who we are. We are defined by our repeated patterns of behaviour. This is described as our character - who we truly are. Through deep and objective analysis, we may come to realise that we have not changed since we were children. Who we are now, is who we were back then. Not in the sense of having the same interests, or the same overt patterns of behaviour; but the same traits are present – only expressing themselves in different ways. Beneath the surface of society's mould; we are who we have always been. If we had distinct ways regarding our behaviour, it is a certainty those traits still show. This, of course is highlighted more if an individual has not made careful and deliberate attempts to override bad habits with new, good habits. By no means is this an insult to the overwhelming majority of us that have not yet managed to adjust. It is more-so recognition and respect for the nature of our individuality.

Here to stay!

The word character has been rooted back to the Greek word Charassein – meaning; 'to engrave'. This supports the idea that our character is something that is carved deeply within. Author, Robert Green, writes about how stress can reveal our flaws. Even the flaws in which we do our best to hide. Green argues that this response to stress is our true character (see fight or flight section). Our first reaction is the closest we get to our truest self. As previously discussed, it is possible for us to program ourselves in order to develop new responses, based on particular cues. Through my observation, one of the most efficient ways to channel this, is through exercise.

One day at the boxing gym, during sparring; my coach told me I need to stop over-thinking and stop waiting for the perfect moment to execute the perfect punch. In that moment, like a punch itself, those words struck me. Throughout my life –including childhood – I can recall many moments of not only being an over-thinker but also being a perfectionist (the two may be related, but that is a conversation for another time). It was a pattern. Just as I had learned in the ring that day, I also had to learn at points throughout my life, that sometimes the perfect moment I was waiting for doesn't arrive. Sometimes we must produce many little moments which create the opportunity to land that perfect punch.

I remember being in my first year of secondary school, there was a subject called design technology. This term in design technology, me and my classmates were given the task of producing a 3D puzzle. Compelled by the prospect of producing something useful, I got right to designing images for my puzzle. I decided to use an image of a character from my favourite cartoon at the time - Dragonball Z. After a few sketches, I asked the teacher and a few classmates for their opinions. Seemingly impressed, their responses filled me with encouragement. However, in my mind, it could still be better. I remember drawing the ears over and over again. Redoing the eyes and the nose. It just had to be perfect; because once it's final, it's final! This was a puzzle that others and I were going to use, therefore it had to look flawless. People had to see that I produced something amazing. We won't get into the root cause of my need for perfection. For now, we are just acknowledging its existence, and the patterns it had created in my life.

Because I sought the perfect aesthetic, I took longer than I should have to complete the drawing. This meant I had less time to work on the part that was more important; the practical part – making the puzzle. With a 'perfect' design but limited time, my puzzle project ended up being a rushed job. Still a decent execution, but not what it could have been had I not been an over-thinking perfectionist. I can recall many other instances in my life where this part of my character had hindered me. It was through exercise, specifically boxing, that this trait was highlighted. Through that same means, is how I was able to channel my over-thinking and become more productive overall. This was also the case with my stubbornness. Although knowledge of my stubborn behaviour preceded any boxing training; it was very much highlighted in training. I soon came to the realisation that a stubborn brain breeds failure in some instances. If I have a failing game plan, I would be a fool if I continued with it - a stubborn fool.

Boxing taught me I had to be less rigid in my ideas, and this mindset translated outside of the ring. My stubbornness is still present, but through the wisdom gained from boxing; I can now express it in other ways - ways that won't hinder my progression. Stubbornness for a good cause is persistence. I am stubborn in finishing tasks that I start. Regardless of how tired I get; I will always push through any exercise - until I break. Through countless rounds on the heavy bag, and countless rounds in the ring, I worked on developing a habit of; what I previously saw as, pre-mature execution. I consciously programmed myself to act, instead of over-thinking. This is a habit that is now present in my everyday life. Who knows; if I didn't override the – once unconscious – habit of false perfectionism with a new habit, maybe even this book never would have been finished. I would still be throwing paper away and starting fresh, 50 years from now.

Think of your more negative traits as an airplane; and your awareness is the pilot. Without a competent pilot, that airplane could go in many directions, before it's inevitable crash. When you have a competent pilot (awareness), you can guide that airplane on a safe journey. And if we use exercise as flight school, we can reach several destinations with that very same airplane. Try not to view character traits as positive or negative. View them in terms of productivity. Is it a hindrance, or a benefit. What you have to do is find the most productive destination to land each airplane.

Through exercise, we can develop patience. Perfecting particular techniques takes time, dedication, and constant practice. Frustration is an easy response, but this would only hinder the progress. In order to perfect the technique – whether in the gym, in the boxing ring, or on the football pitch; patience is mandatory. Transfer the patience you have developed into your tasks at work, or even when dealing with your employer/employees/ co-workers. Channel it into your relationship/marriage. Exercise that patience with your children - they too are learning skills and need to develop patience of their own. Through exercise we can develop resilience. Running that extra mile, or even just doing the number of miles you set out to do, despite feeling fatigued. Whether climbing off the floor to finish a fight, or scoring a last-minute equaliser in a football match after applying consistent pressure - resilience is a natural byproduct of exercise. Use that same resilience to finish your assignment at university despite being mentally overwhelmed. Use that resilience to fight temptation and remain sober after battling with addiction.

Character In Motion

Former cricket player, Shivnarine Chanderpaul, was described by team-mates as 'shy and introverted'. He was a very patient and 'careful' player, which in fact, was consistent with his character. However, it was said –in a surprising manor– that despite his calm, laid-back demeanor, he could be assertive; showing a much tougher character than perceived on field. If we analysed his on-field style closely enough, the 'tough and assertive' traits would not come as a surprise.

Chanderpaul was part of a struggling West Indies team. He was often forced in a situation where the pressure was on him to save the day. This is where his 'careful' patient side was an advantage. He could stand at the crease for hours on end, under immense pressure, but he still managed to maintain the concentration needed in order not to make the slightest mistake. All while resisting the urge to give in to the tricks of the opposition, or to go for glory and 'throw away his wicket'. He exercised these traits, which often helped him to help his team survive. This is indicative of the toughness he possessed. However, despite the good impact that his character had on field, some critics actually called his character into question. One of the criticisms aimed at Chanderpaul was that he was not brave enough to take risks. Not only through his style of play; but it was alleged that he was offered many opportunities to bat higher up in the order – based on his ability – which would have given him the opportunity to produce better scores for himself, and reduce the chances of him having to play the role of the saviour. His decision against batting higher up in the order can be put down to his shy nature – maybe he did not want the spotlight of being one of the main men, so instead, he found comfort hiding in the middle order. Or maybe, deep down he truly was cowardice. The pressure of being relied upon to such extent could have been seen as too much to handle. The survival role may have been viewed as an easier option – if he is successful, all praises to him. But if he fails; it wasn't his fault, he was put in an unfair position. Clever. Maybe in fact, out of all his traits, this highlights his 'careful' risk managing side. Regardless, as one of the few remaining senior players in a West Indies team going through a rebuild, it was inevitable Chanderpaul would have to take on the burden of being a main man. He was eventually made team captain. As with the rest of us, Chanderpaul had a cocktail of character traits. And naturally these traits make themselves visible depending on what we do. When we are forced to demonstrate particular characteristics, we use them on more of a conscious level (e.g. being assertive in the boxing ring). When Chanderpaul was made team captain, he was forced to hone in on his brave, assertive side. This enabled him to channel it at will.

Former team-mate Jimmy Adams spoke on the growth of Chanderpaul: "It was amazing watching, not only your cricket maturing, but also you as a person. From a shy introverted teenager..."

This is the same for all sports; and all exercise in general. A football player can have familiar experiences to those of Chanderpaul. Hiding, or being forced to step up in a make-or-break scenario. A tennis player will have to draw on their mental and physical resilience along with their concentration skills. A boxer will have to be in a constant state of focus; as the consequences are too dire. When exercising, we learn about ourselves. We find out what we are made of. How much do you really push yourself? Do you 'fight' through pain barriers? Are you content with doing the bare minimum? On the days you lack motivation, do you have discipline? It will surface. Exercise and sports, require structure. Structure requires discipline. Discipline incurs responsibility. And responsibility brings forth maturity. When we exercise, the relationship between discipline and results is clear. If we want results, we must be disciplined in our approach.

Use sport or exercise to find out who you are. And then use the sport or exercise to enhance your better, more productive traits. At one point or another we are placed in a situation that challenges us - on the field, in the gym, or in real life. Exercise prepares you for the world.

I agree with the concept of the following quote. But I disagree with it being specific to the sport of cricket:

> *"Cricket is probably the only team sport where players have room to express themselves for who they really are, and personality traits can be identified solely by performances and style of play on the field"*
>
> *- Rishad Dsouza.*

CHAPTER 8

P.A.D.S

Physical wellness is multifaceted, but simple to break down. I like to use the acronym: P.A.D.S - Physical Activity, Diet, Sleep. When these are aligned, our road to wellness is more straightforward. Think of P.A.D.S as a band – but a band with no lead singer. Every member equally as important as the next; and when in harmony, they compose beautiful music. As band manager, your job is to make sure they stay in harmony.

For a professional athlete; it's not that injuries are expected, but it's understood that they come with the territory. Like many others, I'd had the odd minor injury here and there, but fortunately I'd managed to avoid any major ones. But when I did experience my first major injury, I was in a great mental space. I broke my hand, meaning I was likely to be sidelined for months. I could handle the thought of it without any major turn of mood. Even though it was only my hand that was broken, I was told to stay away from all physically activity – including exercise that only involved my legs – to allow the bones to heal properly. I made a promise to myself at the time to make sure that the other band members – diet & sleep – stayed singing in tune. I had sincere intentions of keeping this promise, but I was to find out it was easier said than done. I underestimated the significance of purpose. Physical activity gave me purpose; and when it left, purpose went with it. Bye-bye promise! Unfortunately for me at the time, I didn't have the privilege of reading a book like this one (another doesn't exist). These are realisations I had to come to on my own, so it took a while before I realised what was happening. Being absent from my passion left me void of purpose, and that disrupted the band. I found myself binge-eating junk food and sleeping late. "What's the point of eating healthy, there's no purpose" - probably what my subconscious mind was saying. This continued for a couple of weeks. I blew up to a weight I hadn't been in years. Feeling sluggish during the day due to a lack of sleep and staying in bed well into the afternoon. This was completely out of the ordinary for me.

One afternoon, I was in my bed watching a not-so-exciting TV series, while I scrolled through social media. I was into my 3rd pack of custard cream biscuits, in as many hours. I began to feel physically sick. Definitely because of the number of biscuits I had consumed. As I reached for my water (I still managed to stay health-conscious in that aspect at least), I accidentally dropped the pack of remaining biscuits, leaving crumbs everywhere. Honestly speaking, I don't know if I was more upset by not being able to finish the biscuits, or the fact that I had to get out of bed to clean up my mess. In that moment, like lightning, I was struck with a wake-up call. I jumped up and said, "Forget this!"

"Forget" wasn't the first word I used, but for the sake of this book, I will refrain from the use of profanity. I realised I was becoming lazy due to a lack of purpose, so I gave myself purpose through self-challenge. I needed to get my band singing again, and finding purpose was the best way to start. I neglected "D" and "S" because my passion was solely P.A. I needed to make wellness my passion; and in doing so, it would be easier to keep the other band members singing, even if another was temporarily absent.

This is what I want for you: broaden your passion for wellness. Our mind is at its best when the band is in harmony, but when one temporarily loses its voice, we must keep the others singing. That song will give us peace of mind. Passion is what writes the lyrics, and purpose holds the microphone.

A key takeaway: Be aware of the impact each member has on the band. Be wary of a potential domino effect that a change in structure may have. Let overall wellness be a passion. With that, you will never be void of purpose.

Neglect May Lead to Regret

Despite the severity of the issues that unfolded due to the coronavirus – in the year 2020; some individuals experienced what some may perceive as a silver lining of that grey cloud. Due to the lethal nature of the virus, to function with some normality; some companies allowed their employees to work remotely. Working remotely meant the employee could carry out their regular, or adjusted duties of work from outside of their office or usual place of business - providing their work was able to be carried out with just the use of a laptop or a phone. Surprisingly, some did not experience remote work as advantageous. Rather, a few described it as being counterproductive. This claim was a matter of motivation (the lack of). Similar to what was discussed in the section on habits; for most working people, a cue for productivity was waking up and getting out of bed, then having a shower and putting on their work clothes. Even being in the work environment is a cue itself. For this reason, despite working from home, some followed a specific routine as if they were still going to the office - whether or not they left their house. For those who left their house, it is because they realised a change of environment was necessary for productivity, therefore they chose to work in a library or a coffee shop.

For Daniel – a good friend of mine – this was not the case. Daniel worked in the technology sector, which meant he was able to carry out his work from a laptop. For this reason, he was given the green light to work remotely. Unlike others, he was able to find motivation outside of the office. Because of this, he decided to take full advantage of the opportunity, and he left the United Kingdom. Daniel decided to spend some time in the sunny Caribbean Island of St Lucia. Despite moving to a completely different time zone, his discipline allowed him to stick to the lifestyle routines he developed beforehand. As a genuine fitness fanatic, Daniel would not let two days pass without doing some form of exercise. Being health conscious, he also made a point of staying on top of his diet. He was keen on intermittent fasting (see section on diet). Life could not be better. Eating healthy, exercising, and exploring all the beauty St Lucia had to offer. What had gone unnoticed was his failure to adjust to the time zone. Daniel worked for a UK company. The significance of this is that a UK day starts roughly five or six hours before that of a St Lucian day; therefore, Daniel had to wake up significantly earlier than usual to start work. By the time he finished work – in the late afternoon – it was time for him to make the most out of his day. This usually consisted of beach hopping, town exploration, and exercise; which as a result, led to him having only 3 to 4 hours of sleep nightly. A key member of the group P.A.D.S, was being reduced to a back-up singer. Daniel maintained this for months before returning to the UK, due to issues with his job. On his return, despite no longer waking up extra early for work, he failed to improve the quality of his sleep. In hindsight, maybe waking up extra early for work would have been a better option. Because now that he was no longer working at all at this time, he had no routine whatsoever. After months of a sleep deprived routine, due to work timings, he transitioned into having no routine – consisting of haphazard sleep, due to not working at all. Regardless, Daniel stayed exercising regularly, and for the most part, he stuck to his healthy eating regime.

Looking for a new job can be stressful; and it was. Not so much the process, but the apprehension of not knowing when you will get back the security that comes with having a job. It was overwhelming. For this reason, Daniel decided to let his hair down and enjoy his 34th birthday. A group of us got together for a casual, laid-back day. We did some bowling, and afterwards, we enjoyed some good Mexican food in Central London. After a casual stroll in the city, we called it a night and went our separate ways. The following day was a regular one for me, until it wasn't. I started my day with a calm 5-kilometer run. After a shower and breakfast, I made my way to the gym where I then coached my first 2 sessions of the day. Conveniently, during the break I had before my next session, I received a call from Marvin. Marvin is a mutual friend of Daniel and I. Thinking he was calling to reminisce on the night before, he caught me off guard with the most surprising news. Before I could manage a word; in a down-beat tone, Marvin divulged the news that Daniel had suffered a stroke in the early hours of the morning, and he was in the hospital. Just after celebrating his 34th birthday. In disbelief, my phone almost slipped from my hand as I was processing the news. There was so much to digest at one time. Was Daniel going to be okay? Will he make a full recovery? I thought 34 was too young to have a stroke? Lastly, what brought this on?

On arrival to the hospital, the doctors were unaware of what had happened. They acknowledged the clear distress expressed by Daniel, but after carrying out a CT scan, and an x-ray; they found nothing; expressed their desire to discharge him and reduced his diagnosis to an earache. Thankfully, his brother was still present, and he urged the doctors to continue their checks. Only after an MRI (Magnetic Resonance Imaging) scan, it was revealed that Daniel had suffered a stroke. The scan also revealed the part of his brain that was affected by the stroke. Given his relatively healthy lifestyle, the cause of the stroke was a mystery. The doctors ran several tests to try and find indications. His blood pressure was fine, as were his cholesterol and glucose levels. However, after a detailed probe into Daniel's life, the doctors hypothesised that the prolonged lack of consistent, and quality sleep could have been a major driving force behind the stroke.

The type of stroke Daniel suffered is very rare. So rare, that only 1-4% of all strokes are of this kind. This rare medical disturbance is known as Cerebellar Stroke. This happens when there is restricted blood-flow to the brain; usually because of a clot. The aftereffects of Cerebellar Stroke impacts the survivors' day to day experience. Though the effects can vary, we can't compare the impact that each effect has on different individuals. The fact that every 'body' is different and has unique life experiences; individuals may react differently to the same, or different after-effects. After-effects may include some of the following: Loss of balance and/or coordination, severe dizziness (vertigo), nausea & vomiting, impaired memory, speech problems, double vision, cerebellar cognitive affective syndrome - involving executive function; potentially affecting the mental state and behaviour of a survivor. In Daniel's case, he suffered a loss of balance and coordination, impaired memory, speech impairment, vomiting, and a troubled mental state.

Upon release from the hospital, Daniel described his next few days as fearful. Understandably traumatised; he was reluctant to sleep alone, or even sleep at all – due to the trepidation of re-living what he experienced on the night of his stroke. Daniel was assigned a therapist to help aid his mental state, and thankfully, as time went by, it did just that. In the immediate weeks following his stroke, he was still affected by his impaired memory, in addition to the loss of balance and coordination. At the back of the brain, behind the spinal cord is where your cerebellum is located. Your cerebellum is responsible for balance, coordination, and motor learning. This is why it is not unusual when a disruption in this area – due to a stroke – creates issues with these functions. As previously discussed (see section on autosuggestion), neuroplasticity is the brain's ability to heal itself by forming new neural pathways. Neural pathways are the connections formed by neurons in the brain that allow us to process information. Therefore, to increase our ability to process information, and to improve the quality of our interactions, neuroplasticity is vital. One of the most effective triggers for neuroplasticity, is regular physical exercise.

Multiple studies have shown that people who engage in racket sports have a reduced risk of death, and an increased life expectancy. Cardiovascular benefits, and social benefits are not exclusive to racket sports; therefore, they cannot be the only reasons why playing racket sports may increase life expectancy – in comparison to all other sports. It has been suggested that the reason for this, is that racket sports are centered on coordination; and coordination is an activator of your cerebellum. Keeping your cerebellum functioning well, is a sure way to live a higher quality of life, while reducing the risk of death. Considering this information, Daniel had a plan to get himself back to normal. He asked me if I could do some boxing training with him. At this time, he was not keen on an intense cardiovascular workout. Instead, he wanted the focus of this training to be on coordination, memory, and balance. I designed a program centered around punch combinations and quick reactions. Each punch combination was designed to stimulate and challenge his memory. He not only had to recognise the pattern, he also had to memorise it. However, just recognising and memorising the pattern was not enough. With punch combination work; knowing what to do is only the first step. It then becomes about making your body do what is required. Yes, this takes coordination, but it simultaneously boosts your reaction time. Because for each pattern to be considered as a combination, it must be carried out in a free-flowing manner. A manner that is reasonably paced. Hand-eye coordination, memory, and reflexes/ reaction time were all being stimulated through this one exercise. After just 2 sessions, Daniel claimed to have noticed a substantial difference with his motor functions. I asked him if his recovery would have gone down a similar route if he had chosen to stay at home instead. My reason for asking, was because I was genuinely curious about how the brain would repair itself without external assistance. Daniel told me that in his case, he did not believe that staying at home would have been as impactful. He said that even without sports being involved, just being outdoors would have improved his condition more than staying inside. Being outside, there is a lot happening at one time that the mind has to register. For example, something as simple as crossing a road; you have to assess traffic from different directions, which to most of us, does not seem like a difficult challenge (see section on habit). But when you really analyse the need to activate multiple motor processes at once, you begin to understand the amount of concentration that is required. A lot is happening simultaneously. You must visually watch traffic from multiple directions, whilst also listening to it, as a way of sensing danger – all while having to anticipate what some drivers may or may not do.

In Daniel's unique experience, the boxing training was an amplified version of crossing a road. With a lot happening at one time, it triggered the need of concurrent motor functioning. Remembering the right punches – and throwing them at the right time, anticipating and avoiding incoming hits coming back towards him, moving forward, backwards, and side to side – while maintaining the correct posture needed for boxing. When Daniel returned to playing football with his friends again, he reiterated this sentiment. Feet-eye coordination, running, anticipation and visual scanning, are all examples of the multiple, motor functions required at one moment. The benefits of staying active through sport had transferred into his day-to-day life, however. With each day he was getting sharper; and by engaging his brain in these ways, he started to also notice an improvement with his memory. As a result of these realisations, Daniel's confidence started to grow.

Sports in particular requires interaction, and Daniel claims that the social aspect had also helped him to overcome his anxiety – which ironically, helped him to sleep better. Keeping with the theme of irony, quality sleep is also an agent that triggers neuroplasticity - which as we discussed, is vital in the recovery process post-stroke. Daniel's story is a clear demonstration of the full circle regarding sleep. It was his prolonged lack of quality sleep that led to his major health disruption. But quality sleep is what played a significant role in his road to recovery.

Create your own

Note; regarding the sport of boxing, there are only 6 punches. These punches are Jab (1), cross (2), left-hook (3), right-hook (4), left-uppercut (5), right-uppercut (6). Even if you are alone, you can practice these punches. There are plenty of tutorials online that can teach you how to properly execute each punch. But what you can do, if you want to improve your memory, focus, and co-ordination; is create a few combinations by using some or all of these punches. For example; 6-3-2, or; 1-2-3-4. Memorise these self-created combinations and spend a few minutes each day practicing them. You will find stimulation in the challenge, but you will benefit greatly from the action.

Quality over quantity

Good sleep is essential for the overall wellbeing of our bodies and minds. It is often neglected due to our lack of understanding about its importance. Whatever lifestyle we choose to live, quality sleep is a vital component.

We generally live our lives with the idea that sleep is as simple as going to bed when we are tired and waking up when we are recharged. The modern world, however, presents many complex lifestyles. And because of this, a simplistic approach towards sleep is hardly practical. For many of us we are far removed from the times when our lifestyle was in sync with our body's behavioral patterns. Once upon a time; we would rise as the sun rose and sleep not long after it went down, but life in the modern world makes this more difficult.

The average day of 2 individuals may hardly look the same. Even if they work the same job, their lives outside of work may be different. The structure of, or obligations to one's family may be a factor, as well as how one's leisure preferences would come into play. Take Daniel for instance. He had colleagues with the same job role, some of which may have also decided to work from the Caribbean. But Daniel's preferences for sightseeing and general exploration is what dictated how he managed his time – and how you manage your time will greatly influence the structure of your sleep. Imagine the differences in sleeping patterns between those with different shifts, different jobs, and different interests outside of work. In most societies in the past this may have not been a factor; but certainly today, the attainment of quality sleep requires an intentional approach. Our lifestyle is an umbrella, with many sub-factors beneath it. With modern times has come new structures and conditions for us to live in. Beyond new structures, modern times has also brought about new technology – which is extremely influential in our behaviours that lead to the quality of sleep we manage. For example, take a device such as a tablet. It is easy to be distracted and lose track of time while being engrossed in it – which can lead to getting less sleep. But even from a scientific perspective, these devices are against our greater interests. In his book 'sleep smarter', Shawn Stevenson breaks down several ways – beyond time management – that the quality of our sleep is influenced.

Understand the difference between length of sleep and quality of sleep. It's possible to have 8 hours of non-interrupted sleep, and that sleep be of poor quality. A sleep cycle is the pattern of stages our bodies go through whilst asleep. Those that manage to get 8 hours of sleep have roughly 5 sleep cycles – given that each sleep cycle lasts between 80 to 120 minutes. The cycles begin the moment you fall asleep, and end the moment you

wake. There are 4 stages that make up a cycle of sleep. For a good quality of sleep to be achieved, we must spend a specific length of time in each of the 4 stages. Out of the 4, one of these stages is known as 'rapid eye movement' (REM); whereas the other 3 all fall into the category of NREM (non-rapid eye movement). Although they fall into the same category, each stage serves a different purpose, thus requires a different length of time.

The 4 stages are as follows:

1. N1 - This is the first stage of NREM. It is the stage we enter as we initially fall asleep; thus, why it is also referred to as 'stage 1 sleep'. N1 does not last for long, its purpose is to act as a vehicle to take you from wakefulness to sleep. The brain starts to slow down – our brainwaves go from alpha waves (neural oscillations in the frequency range of 8-12Hz) to theta waves (a lower frequency

range of 4 - 8Hz). During N1 your body starts to slow down - your muscles begin to relax and your body temperature starts to fall. At this point the body is not completely relaxed, therefore you can be easily woken. There is still slow, side to side eye movement. N1 accounts for roughly 5% of TST (total sleep time), and when uninterrupted, people quickly move into the 2nd stage of sleep.

2. N2 - The 2nd stage of NREM. During N2; your body temperature falls further, your muscles relax more, your breathing and heart rate also decrease, and your eye movement completely stops. Your brain waves display a new pattern with short bursts of activity. Though you are still susceptible to being easily awakened, these short bursts help prevent it. N2 is vital because if interrupted, it may negatively impact your ability to commit new skills to your memory. Despite lasting approximately 25 minutes in your first cycle, N2 gets longer with each sleep cycle and eventually accounts for roughly 50% of TST.
3. N3 - Out of the 3 stages of NREM, N3 is where we experience the deepest sleep. Our brain waves are now in the form of what is known as delta waves – signals with lower frequencies and higher amplitudes. Immune system strengthening, tissue growth and repair, and cell regeneration all occur during N3 stage of sleep. By this time, your body is completely relaxed, and it is very difficult to be woken up. N3 lasts between 20-40 minutes and accounts for roughly 20% of TST.
4. Rapid eye movement (REM) - Similar to N2, REM length increases with each cycle during sleep, with the last cycle lasting roughly 10 minutes. Brain activity during REM is similar to when you are awake, and coincidentally, REM is the stage which people tend to randomly wake up. This stage hosts our dreams, and it makes up about 25% of our TST. Lack of REM sleep can be the cause of memory issues.

This may be a case of stating the obvious; light and darkness have a strong influence on our circadian timing system (sleep cycles). The relationship is complex. The amount of sunlight you receive during the day, and at specific times of the day, directly impacts how good of a sleep you manage. Our bodies release specific hormones at specific times of the day. These hormones, in conjunction with our CTS (circadian timing system) assist in controlling our digestion, immune system, blood pressure, fat utilisation, appetite, and mental energy. The hypothalamus in the brain is home to a small group of nerve cells known as suprachiasmatic nucleus. These nerve cells are what regulates our CTS. Due to its control of our hunger, our thirst, energy levels, and our body temperature, the hypothalamus is viewed as the master gland for our hormonal system. This master gland, along with all corresponding glands and organs, are triggered by light. Light exposure, namely sunlight, signals to the body to produce substantial levels of what is known as daytime hormones. These daytime hormones together with neurotransmitters that are also produced, regulates our biological clocks. Serotonin is a neurotransmitter that assists in bringing the feeling of happiness. This is why many antidepressant drugs are designed to spike our serotonin levels. Light exposure brings about a natural influence on our serotonin. Too little sunlight during the day, or too much artificial light in the evening will have a negative impact on how our bodies produce this important neurotransmitter.

When sleep is not optimal, we risk disrupting the function of our adrenal gland. This will create a cycle because a disrupted adrenal gland will be a key reason as to why your sleep will continue to be of poor quality. The adrenal gland is responsible for the production of cortisol – a stress hormone – which when under or over produced, has a negative impact on our cycle of sleep. Cortisol is the reason you are able to attain alertness, strength, focus, and vitality upon waking up in the morning. Your adrenal produces it for this purpose and as the day goes on, your cortisol levels decrease. This cortisol rhythm prepares you for a quality sleep. An effective means of regulating this rhythm is by getting daytime exposure to sunlight. Sunlight exposure boosts cortisol levels, creating the tone for an optimal rhythm. Melatonin is a hormone produced by the pineal gland, as a response to darkness. When melatonin levels are up, cortisol levels are down. And when cortisol levels are up, melatonin levels are down. Melatonin production aids us in getting a good quality sleep, as do cortisol levels. However, the timing of the production of these hormones is vital. If sunlight exposure spikes our cortisol, and cortisol is responsible for energy and alertness, it would be wise to expose ourselves to as much daytime sunlight as possible. Similarly, if darkness spikes our melatonin, and melatonin encourages a state of restfulness, it would be beneficial for us to avoid lights during the evening. When we are exposed to too much light in the evening, we encourage further production of cortisol; leading to more energy and alertness within ourselves. Light is a blocker of melatonin production; therefore when

we expose ourselves to light – particularly sunlight – during the day, the possibility of being in a state of quiet wakefulness is significantly reduced.

During the winter, or year-round in certain regions; it may be difficult to get natural light exposure during the day. However, even on overcast days, the sun rays still make it through the clouds – which is why we experience daytime. These sun rays are enough to have a positive influence on your hormonal function. Therefore, it is important that we find time to go outside early in the day to expose ourselves to as much of it as possible. Between the hours of 10pm - 2am is when we experience our most advantageous hormone secretions. This is why being asleep during these hours is beneficial. HGH (human growth hormone), known as the youth hormone, is one of a few secreted. This allows our bodies to strengthen, repair, and rejuvenate. Reducing the chances of this secretion can speed up the process of aging.

Below is a table demonstrating factors that negatively affect our sleep; and the ways that we can negate these factors.

Problem	Reason	Advice
Technological "smart" devices	Devices such as tablets, smartphones, televisions – all give off what is known as blue light. This blue light tricks the brain into thinking it is currently daytime; which disrupts melatonin production.	• Cut screen time – experts recommend minimum of 3 hours before bed. If unavoidable, there are several apps available for download that can block the blue light being emitted by your device. • Blue light blocking glasses. • Use dim, red lights
Caffeine	Stimulates nervous system and encourages adrenal glands to produce cortisol and adrenaline. This is bound to disrupt your sleep cycle; and the disruption of your cycle will make you crave more caffeine – creating an ongoing cycle.	• Create a caffeine curfew. • Avoid caffeine within 6 hours of your bedtime. • Intake as close to your wake-up period as possible.

Bad bacteria in the gut	• 95% of serotonin in the body is located in the gut. • Serotonin plays a vital role in the secretion of melatonin. The gut itself produces 400 times more melatonin than what is produced by the pineal gland. • Just like the brain, our gut is made up of tissue. • Vagus nerve is what connects your gut to your brain – making interactions with your heart, lungs, and other organs along the way. • Gut is full of friendly and unfriendly bacteria. When you sleep poorly, the bad bacteria take control of your gut, thus, your brain, potentially causing sleep deprivation. • Sleep deprivation leads to over-eating and poorer food choices. This results in the continuous reign of bad bacteria in the gut.	**Avoid**: • Agricultural chemicals such as pesticides. • Processed foods. • Chemical preservatives/food additives. • Chlorinated water. • Irregular or constant intake of antibiotics.

Specific house plants and air purifiers are other ways of attaining quality sleep. Plants such as lavender, jasmine, snake plant, pothos, aloe vera, are all known to improve sleep quality.

Eat To Live

Moses Ben Maimon – also known as 'Maimonides', was a rabbi and philosopher. He lived during the 12th and 13th century. Maimonides was considered a man of wisdom; and a lot of such wisdom, he applied to physical wellness. His overall fondness of wellness came in the face of tragedy. His wife unfortunately lost her life while birthing their child. It was after that tragic moment that Maimonides became meticulous in his approach towards holistic health. He spent years studying what works best for, and what is bad for the human body. His observations were broad. He covered behavioural patterns concerning physical activity, diet, and sleep – or lack of. Regarding dietary concerns; Maimonides was direct, and uncomplicated in his advice. He recommended the following approach: "Be strict with portion sizes. Over-eating is poison to the body."

What we put into our body is also closely related to the quality of sleep we manage.

Below is a table detailing the types of nutrients which may improve sleep quality.

Nutrient	Foods to find it
Calcium: disturbances in REM is linked to calcium deficiency.	Kale, collard greens, sardines, sea vegetables, sesame seeds.
Selenium: positively boosts immune system and thyroid function. Deficiency can cause sleep abnormalities.	Brazil nuts, sunflower seeds, beet, oysters, chicken, cremini mushrooms.

Vitamin C: regulates neurotransmitters. Deficiency may affect duration and quality of sleep.	Amla berry, acerola cherry, bell peppers, leafy green vegetables, kiwi, strawberry, citrus fruits, papaya.
Potassium: aids muscle and nerve function. Deficiency can cause spasms.	Leafy green vegetables, potato, broccoli, cremini mushrooms, avocado, baked beans.
Vitamin D: deficiency can increase the risk of sleep disorders.	Salmon, tuna, mackerel, oysters. The best source of vitamin D is natural sunlight.
Tryptophan: the body uses this amino acid to produce serotonin.	Turkey, chicken, eggs, sweet potato, banana, chia seeds, hemp seeds, pumpkin seeds, almonds, leafy green vegetables.
Omega 3: this is a fatty acid that contributes to a deeper, more restful sleep.	Chia seeds, pumpkin seeds, hemp seeds, walnuts, flax seeds, salmon.
Melatonin: essential for a quality sleep.	Tart cherries (food source with the highest amount), pineapple, banana, tomato, oranges.
Vitamin B: relaxes the nervous system.	Banana, cashew nuts, peanut butter, almonds, avocado, tomato, spinach, fish, sweet potato, eggs.

P.A.D.S is the greatest example of what a team should be. Though demonstrating great teamwork, each member pulls its own weight. As we can see in the table above, nutrients that play a significant role in 'S' can be attained through 'D'. Good 'S' puts us in a position to incorporate sufficient 'P.A'. And good 'P.A' also contributes to quality 'S'. However, neither 'P.A' or 'S 'are maximised to their greatest potential without the assistance of quality 'D'.

P.A.D.S is the circle of wellness. To look past it is to do ourselves a disservice.

Structure In Diet

A lot of the time, the external reflects the internal; and the state of the internal is largely determined by our eating habits. If I were to do a road trip, I'd be sure to fill my vehicle with quality gas, and enough of it. The type of vehicle, and the desired destination will determine the type of fuel required (see T1 for an overview). But beyond the type of fuel – in this case food – modern and ancient times boast a variety of methods that may be used to arrive at the destination of wellness. Every 'body' is different, one size doesn't fit all. That's why it's better to explore different methods before committing.

Practiced in many cultures – ancient and modern – one popular dietary practice is intermittent fasting. Intermittent fasting is a food cycle where the individual schedules a time for voluntary fasting and non-fasting. There are many variations of this. A popular and one of the least difficult types of intermittent fasting is known as 16/8. The 16/8 method is scheduled over a period of 24 hours (a day); which provides a simple structure. Out of the 24 hours, 16 of them will be without food (voluntary fasting), leaving an 8-hour window for consumption. This may seem more difficult than it is. When we factor in the number of hours we (should) sleep, the window of voluntary fasting is shorter. This is how many people who practice 16/8 operate. If I were doing 16/8 and i wake up at 8am, I could wait until 12pm before having my first meal (consuming water up until that point). My cut off time for food would be 8pm. I'd have sufficient time to eat during my window; giving my body what it requires, whilst leaving adequate time for the organs and cells to repair during the night. Some reasons why people may decide to adopt intermittent fasting could be for weight loss, to lower blood sugar levels, better gut health, and to reduce inflammation.

Some studies have suggested that intermittent fasting has an impact on all of the above.

However, the correlation shown in these studies do not necessarily show causation. Regarding weight loss, the argument can be made that people who do intermittent fasting tend to reduce their calorie intake or simply eat healthier meals than usual. As a result, they will lose weight. To reduce your calorie intake, intermittent fasting is not a requirement. Let's not ignore the importance of structure. Using myself as an example, the times that I've practiced intermittent fasting; I made a conscious decision to eat healthier. It had a snowball effect. Making one healthier step led me to making another. I'm aware that this won't be the case for everyone.

The first type of intermittent fasting that I attempted was the 5:2. With this structure, I would eat as normal for 5 days (for me, in a row) and reduce my calorie intake on the other 2 days. It sounded good in theory, but in reality, I found myself over-eating during the 5 days as a way of compensating for the caloric reduction on the other 2. this type of intermittent fasting was not effective for me, which is the reason i switched to another type. I'm aware that the over-compensating I was doing is what some others may do when practicing the 16:8. This is why it's necessary to explore and figure out what works best for you.

Daily patterns provide us with structure. And this structure – regarding our diet – will positively influence our circadian rhythm. When our mealtimes are consistent it boosts our metabolism, which aids weight management. Studies show how disrupting the process of regular mealtimes can increase the risk of weight gain and other health issues. Irregular mealtimes have been shown to lead to high blood pressure, obesity, and type 2 diabetes. One study had one group consume more calories overall, whilst sticking to the same mealtimes each day. Whereas the other group consumed less calories but had an inconsistent eating schedule. The first group had better insulin and cholesterol levels, and were less obese, despite consuming more calories. Structure is key!

Below is a table showing various ways we can make our diet healthier. Along with each method, I have included both advantages and disadvantages.

Method	Advantage(s)	Disadvantage(s)
Water fasting: consuming nothing but water for an extended period. Commonly practiced between 24-48 hours.	• Weight loss • Decreased blood pressure • Mental resilience	• Can potentially worsen diabetes • Electrolyte imbalance • Muscle loss • Fatigue • Possible increased • anxiety or irritability
Calorie deficit: either exercise to burn more calories, or limit calorie intake with food. Or both.	• Weight loss • Improved body composition • Improved insulin • sensitivity • Reduced inflammation • Reduced risk of chronic disease	• When in calorie deficit, the body breaks down fat for energy which has the potential to cause gallstones • Risk of causing malnutrition • Low energy
Juice diet: involves only consuming juices from fruits and vegetables.	• Increased nutrition intake • Improved heart health • Improved kidney function • Improved hydration • Weight loss	• Low calorie intake • Potentially not enough protein or fat
Intermittent fasting	• Weight loss • Structure • Improved brain function	• Hunger • Fatigue • May cause binge eating

"Let food be thy medicine, and medicine be thy food" - Hippocrates

Understanding P.A

Fuelling your body in the correct way will lead to feeling better all round. Particularly, it impacts how effectively we exercise. Regardless of differences between our goals, it is always important to make exercise as efficient as possible so that we can achieve them. This efficiency is expressed differently depending on the individual goal. And this goal, will determine the type of exercise carried out. To understand the best exercises for our goals, we must understand how different exercises generate different reactions.

Adenosine triphosphate (ATP) is a molecule that carries energy for the purpose of powering our cells. It is the primary source of energy for a lot of our biological functions, and one of the ways it is made is by a breakdown of the food we consume. When we consume foods high in protein (meat, fish, dairy, eggs, legumes, nuts, seeds), our bodies break this protein down to form a compound known as amino acids. Another compound known as glucose is produced by the breakdown of carbohydrates. Some examples of high carbohydrate foods are as follows: pasta, rice, potato, fruit, vegetables. The more of these foods we eat is the higher the concentration of glucose we will produce. Fatty acids are what the body produces when we consume food that contains a high level of fat. Food such as; oils, salmon, avocado, dairy. When these compounds – amino acids, glucose, fatty acids – are produced, they are then absorbed into the blood and carried to various cells. Once in the cells, these compounds then help to produce ATP. For ATP to now be supplied to the necessary cells throughout the body, we rely on what are known as energy systems.

Energy systems are biochemical processes that our bodies use to produce energy during exercise. Performance coach Josh Swaray describes energy systems as a type of bank. "A place your body withdraws currency (energy) in order to effectively function." physical activity causes the heart rate to elevate; and the rate of elevation will determine which account (energy system) you will withdraw from. The two energy systems commonly mentioned in the world of exercise are; aerobic system, anaerobic system. The aerobic system provides energy for low or medium intensity activities

– lasting anywhere between 2 minutes to a few hours. This system is the bank that endurance athletes mainly withdraw from.

The table below shows a few examples of aerobic activities, along with some of the benefits.

Aerobic activity	Benefits
Jogging/long runs (less than 75% of maximum speed)	Improves cardiovascular fitness. Does not necessarily require equipment.
Cycling - steady paced	Low impact.
Swimming	Full body, joint relief, cardiovascular fitness.
Brisk walking	Simple and effective way to improve endurance and increase heart rate.
Skipping (jump rope)	Improves cardio and coordination.
Dancing	Fun, whilst increasing heart rate.

The word aerobic means "in the presence of oxygen", therefore aerobic training is any form of training where the intake of oxygen is required. When this is the case, it is usually because the exercise is completed over a sustained period. Aerobic training is usually executed at a steady pace, without any pronounced spikes of energy use. The most emphasised benefit of aerobic training is improved cardiovascular health. With improved cardiovascular health our day-to-day tasks are less draining, the quality of life is better, and studies show that it can lead to an improved mental condition. This is something that applies not only to sports people, but also to the everyday person that incorporates aerobic training into their lifestyle.

Type 1 muscle fibers (slow twitch fibers) are endurance-oriented and contain cells that are considerably smaller than those found in Type 2 fibers (fast twitch fibers). Fast twitch fibers are engaged during anaerobic training, and they fatigue quicker than slow twitch fibers. These Type 2 (fast twitch) fibers easily achieve muscle growth; therefore, if the goal is to grow your muscles, these fast twitch fibers must be engaged. Anaerobic training is the only door to the house of muscle growth.

Some of the most effective anaerobic training methods are as follows:

- Strength training – exercising with heavier loads (weights).
- Explosive training – lighter weights with explosive tempos.
- Plyometric training – E.g. explosive box jumps, burpees, forward hops, lunge jumps, medicine ball throws.
- Resistance training – E.g. calisthenics (pull ups, push-ups, plank), band exercises, hill sprints.

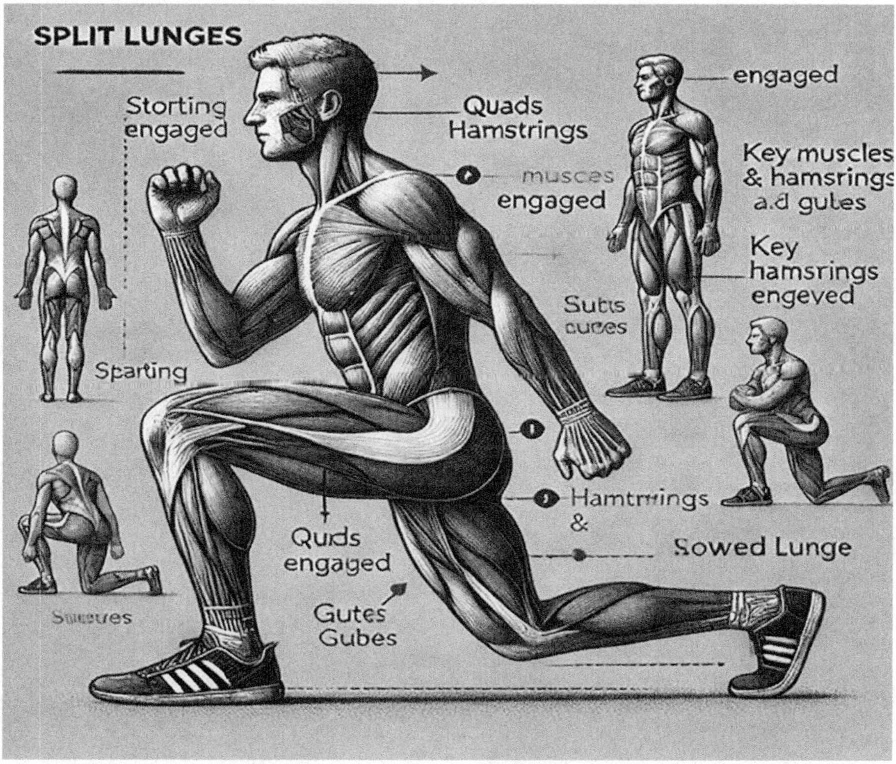

CHAPTER 9

The long run

If you value your dream, you will value your team.

There is no limit on how late in life someone can begin to exercise. Nor should there be any restriction on how early. For every age, there is something that can be done. But it's definitely a matter of the earlier the better. Through sport and exercise, we develop important traits. And these traits can serve us throughout our lives. Therefore, the earlier these traits are developed, the better.

Boxing is one of a few individual sports. It's often referred to as "the loneliest sport in the world". Though this is the case, it still takes a team for the individual to be successful. Every boxer needs a coaching team, but beyond that, they all benefit from training partners that help push them. Whether that be sparring partners, or others joining in with the sprint sessions, training partners contribute to the progression of the individual. I remember when I was an amateur boxer training for a tournament. Me and 5 of my stable mates were entered this particular time. At this stage, we hadn't known each other for a long time. But being on a joint mission is what bonded us. Because of how lonely the sport gets, boxers long for understanding. People may understand boxing from the outside, but they will never truly grasp the experience. This is why for boxers; being around each other brings relatability. And that relatability; founded on a mutual respect, brings a unique type of bond. When training together, it's about much more than having a bond. It becomes a duty. They have a responsibility to push one another. Even by pushing themselves to the limit, they are pushing each other; because resilient energy is infectious. For us that were training for this tournament, we also had a responsibility to represent our gym in the best way we could. Just like working for a company or even being in a romantic relationship; the greater good is beyond you as an individual. This is a type of accountability that can help any individual grow. The sacrifice of your comfort for the greater good, is the key to success.

Beyond the obvious competitive goals; sport demonstrates responsibility, accountability, and sacrifice. In terms of football, each team begins a game with 11 players on the field. Each player is placed in a position they are specially equipped for. And depending on pre-game tactics, they each have their own roles. Legendary football coach Louis Van Gaal, when speaking on the principles he imbeds in his teams, says; "Each player needs to know where he has to be, and that is why there needs to be mutual understanding because you need absolute discipline." It is the job of the striker to score goals, and it is the job of the 'keeper to help his team prevent goals. If a team is to be successful, it needs to be exactly that – a team. To meet the overall goal, players must put their ego to the side and play their role. Having 11 individuals on the same side isn't enough to call them a team. Technically, and in theory, yes. But in reality, to be a team, there must be 'chemistry'. This 'chemistry' is a result of the individuals understanding the roles they have to play. The left-sided defender shouldn't be focused on being the one to score the goals – unless opportunity presents itself. His/her job should be to nullify the efforts of the oppositions right-sided winger. Despite the differences in roles between the players, Van Gaal says that the 'philosophy' must always remain. At a stage in his career, he was the manager of the biggest football club in England – Manchester United. During a press conference after a victory, Van Gaal was confronted with a question regarding the alleged defensive vulnerability of his team. His response: "It's not about the defenders; the whole team defend." That statement perfectly describes his 'philosophy' – regardless of individual roles, the players defend as a team, and attack as a team. Removing individual blame when a goal is conceded, means there is no hiding place for any player when things go wrong. They are all responsible, and in the same sense, they are all praised when things go to plan. It is a team effort – an incentive to always give 100%

Manchester United is not only the biggest club in England, but one of the biggest sporting clubs on the planet. In the year 1999, they famously won what is known in football as a treble. This is the case of a team winning the 3 biggest trophies in a single season. In this particular season, the players had to use their "fighting spirit and never say die mentality" on numerous occasions, scoring last gasp winning goals. Never giving up was a theme of their season – something that trickled down from the coaching staff to the players, and even to the fans. The mentality was imbedded by their leader, the manager at the time – Sir Alex Ferguson. Even if resilience wasn't in the natural make-up of a player; they developed it along the way. They had no choice but to; partly because of the responsibility they had for one another. You had to rise a level, and a strong leader – in this instance, the team captain Roy Keane – helps to raise the standard. Bold, fearless, relentless, and skillful, Keane always led by example on the pitch. A stand-out game of his that season came in the UEFA Champions League semi-final. Battling against some of football's greatest ever midfield players, Roy Keane excelled – even scoring a goal in the process. Manchester United went on to win the game – securing a place in the final – after being in a losing position. But unfortunately for Keane, due to a disciplinary issue in the game, he was banned from playing in the final. This meant the team would be without their 2 best midfield players for the final (Paul Scholes) was also suspended. The other players had to now take responsibility and step up. That's exactly what they did! Despite being in a losing position for most of the game, Manchester United once again showed their resilience. They scored 2 goals in the last minute of the match to win the game, and the Champions League. At one point, even the goal-keeper was in the opposition box trying to help his team to score. They did all they could to fight for each other. Quitting would have been easy. Blaming the fact their 2 best players were absent would have been easy.

In the same season, they experienced many tests. Tests that their mentality got them through. Notably in the FA Cup semi-final, when they went down to 10-men against their fierce rivals. Disadvantaged, against all odds, their fighting spirit carried them through. Because once again, the players fought for each other. The interesting part about that for me is that not all the players within that team got along with each other. But they understood the overall goal. Andrew Cole and Teddy Sheringham famously had issues between them. But nothing was above the team winning.

Killing the ego and putting team success over individual feuds, showing resilience to win from losing positions, stepping up when your best players are missing, fighting hard when going down to 10 men, showing respect for authority and following the lead of competent leaders (captain & manager), going above and beyond your role as a 'keeper to help your team score; are all great attributes that can be attained through playing sport – not limited to football. Below are some examples of how these attributes can help you in different parts of your life.

Professionally:

– Good mood in the workplace; less chance of depression, meaning the staff are more likely to get along.
– Chemistry; sport creates a bond between its participants. This bond can be carried into the workplace.

– Better health; employees will miss less workdays because of illness, therefore there is potential for increased productivity.
– Responsibility; team work is about constant awareness of the overall goal, and trying to reach it by any means. Even if it means going beyond your role.
– Respect for authority; learning to trust your leader.

Socially:

– Making friends/building community; all forms of exercise are known to encourage bonding. It's a universal language we can all speak to some degree. Playing football in the park with strangers, walking groups, running clubs, dance classes – exercise unites us in a joyful way.
– Confidence; Women, and men, face a lot of pressure regarding body image. Though there may not be immediate physical changes; the mental benefits experienced also comes with confidence. Feeling productive, feeling fitter & stronger, and having less anxiety are all benefits to be gained.
– Recognition; if recognition is what's desired, this will be a possibility when physical progress is made. Particularly in the age of social media.

Academically:

– Enhanced focus; exercise boosts focus.
– Group work; team sport can prepare students for a group setting in which each member has a responsibility to fulfil their role.
– Resilience/drive; sport can teach an individual about finishing what they start.
– Improved grades; refer to section on 'zero hour P.E'.
– Authority; respecting authority figures during team sport could translate into students respecting their teachers – if they lacked that previously.

Romantically:

– Studies support the claim that couples who train together, stay together (mentioned later in this chapter). A few of the reasons given for this are as follows:

- A common goal with your partner increases your bond.
- A mental outlet is being had by both parties.
- Obtaining desired body goals can increase physical attraction.
- Quality time.
- Responsibility; understanding you have a role, and a responsibility to the overall goal – the success of the relationship.
- Increased comfort – during exercise we are in a vulnerable state. Exposing ourselves in this way to our partner brings a new level of comfort, thus increased trust.

Sport and exercise are the greatest ways to give yourself, your friends, and even your children great character traits. These traits will serve them through many walks of their lives. Get involved and get great!

No choice but to endure!

Life itself can be metaphorised as a marathon, a long run. And aspects within life can too be described that way. In the case of wellness, it is the lifestyle that is a marathon. When we have wellness goals, we can approach them in a manner reminiscent of climbing a mountain. To climb, we need particular tools (P.A.D.S). When we reach our target, if we were to dispose of the tools that we used to take us there – a harness for example, it would be nearly impossible to climb any further. Even if we had no desire to go any further; to stay at a particular level, we would still need equipment to keep us alive. Now you ask; "but what if we got to the top of the mountain?" And that is where the comparison ends, because with wellness, there is no top. We must always remember the need for our tools, or we risk falling from whichever point we are on that mountain.

Channel your inner Shackleton – we all have it!

Polar explorer Ernest Shackleton experienced many voyages, but he is highly regarded for one particular expedition – the Imperial Trans-Antarctic Expedition. After his loss in the race to the south pole, Shackleton was determined to make the first land crossing of the Antarctic continent. More than a simple voyage, this journey was one of struggle and stress, but also courage and conviction. When we analyse this story, we can see how comparable it is to our individual journey towards wellness. With unexpected challenges, mental struggles, and sacrifice; just like Ernest Shackleton's voyage, we must be adaptable, resilient, and efficient in using the right tools in order to succeed.

The ship 'Endurance' was designed by Ole Aanderud Larsen, and was constructed meticulously, with the purpose of being strong and durable. 140 feet long, Endurance was approximated to weigh 340 tons. At the time of its launch in 1912, it was possibly the strongest ship constructed to date. In January of 1914, Shackleton purchased the ship which, was originally named 'Polaris'. Once purchased, he renamed the ship to Endurance – in honour of his family motto 'Fortitude Vincimus', which means 'by endurance we conquer' – very fitting! Ernest Shackleton spent months making slight alterations to the ship, gathering a crew, and adding equipment; notably three relatively small ship boats. Finally ready, Endurance left London in August of 1914, reaching the whaling station in South Georgia on November 5th, before setting sail for Antarctica a month later. A voyage consisting of 27 men, and around 100 dogs (purchased by Shackleton for the purpose of pulling the sleds that carried supplies) was under way. After just 2 days, the ship met with polar pack ice and was forced to slow its pace from then on. Despite now being relatively close to its next destination, Endurance was met with further obstacles. Worsening weather conditions and heavy pack ice forced Endurance to take shelter under a large iceberg for 2 days. The easing weather conditions allowed the ship to restart its journey; but only briefly, because once again, it was met with heavy pack ice. This time, the men decided to proceed and maneuver through the ice. This attempt was a failure. The extremely heavy wind indurated the ice from the sea against the land, which meant there was nothing that could be done, other than to wait and hope for an opposing wind. A wind strong enough to undo what this fierce wind had caused. Despite the trouble, Shackleton maintained his high energy and enthusiasm, in hope that his mood continued to rub off on his crew. He valued discipline, thus made sure he and his crew stuck to a routine. This aided the mood. Shackleton believed that if everyone was in high spirits, it would be easier for all to be on the same page – and being on the same page makes progress a simpler process.

January 20th, 1915; serious pressure caused Endurance to become trapped. Shackleton needed to be pro-active and he did this by working together with his crew to manually move the ship from the ice into the water. After more than a month trying, the men finally gave up and accepted the reality which was that the ship at that moment was merely a winter station. From time to time, the ship would drift with no direction, but the men remained patient in hope that they would eventually regain control of the situation. The game of patience – in this case – was one that required distraction. The men would play football on the ice to keep their spirits up. And eventually, the once sled dogs, had become pets. After noticing the ice closing in and surrounding the ship, the men – with their shovels – decided to try once more to move the ice manually. Another attempt that was met with failure; and once more, the men accepted that they had no choice but to wait it out. The harsh weather had continued for months. It was now July, and the pressure had become overwhelming. The ship Endurance was damaged beyond repair! The men were stranded, trapped now for 7 months, running low on supplies, 1200 miles from civilisation, with no outside communication or help. This was now a test of their physical, and mental resolve.

On October 18th, a wave of pressure caused the ship to tip over, all within a matter of seconds. Tilted at 30 degrees, Endurance wasn't only bent and twisted, it was now leaking. The men used blankets in an attempt to contain the leaks. All to no success – they were forced to abandon the ship just 9 days later. Shackleton knew that despite how he felt; if he remained calm, his men would notice this and remain calm themselves. Up to this point, despite the previous troubles, morale was initially high. Wherever the men attempted to march, they were blocked by ice. Though having the 3 wooden lifeboats from the ship, the men had to wait to be closer to land before they could make use of them. Eventually, supplies ran low, and the crew – including the dogs – were surviving off the penguin and seal meat that they hunted. They were forced to ration; each man having 1 biscuit for lunch, and 3 lumps of sugar each day.

The date was 30th March 1916, and all supplies are completely finished – not a seal or penguin in sight. Shackleton made the tough decision to kill and eat the dogs that they grew to love. This also lessened the burden that the men had in looking after the dogs. By April 9th, the storms were monstrous, and the men were now a few days in with no sleep. With each day came 17 hours of darkness, and with that, a promise of unpredictability. Finally, after 16 months in ruin; the men reached the land of Elephant Island and enjoyed their first bit of food after going 3 days without. Then on April 24th, 1916, Shackleton made the brave decision to leave 22 of his men behind while he and 5 others faced the vicious sea on 1 of the tiny wooden boats – in an attempt to find a whaling station on South Georgia Island. Predictably; on this quest, his troubles continued. If Shackleton and his men weren't being hit by enormous waves, it was gale wind hitting them. After 2 weeks of battling through, the 6 men spotted South Georgia coast, and spent the next 2 days attempting to land on shore. When they finally reached the shore, Shackleton realised they landed on the wrong side of the island – opposite to where the whaling station was located. And just their luck; what was in their way? glaciers and mountains! Glaciers and mountains that had never been crossed before. After all they had been through prior to this moment, it would have been understandable to fall at the challenge, but the men welcomed it. Despite being underprepared for this crossing, they were at least equipped with rope. 3 of the men were feeling too weak to make this trip, so it was agreed they'd stay behind. Shackleton and the 2 others put screws into their shoes for added grip, and they began to trek.

Despite being delayed at first due to a storm, the trio managed to climb approximately 3000 feet after the first day. It was now vital that they got to the bottom of this hill before the sky got dark. With limited time, a brave decision was made. Standing at the top of this steep hill, unbeknown to what was waiting at the bottom, the men had no time to be tentative. They coiled their rope down, sat on it, put their arms around each other's waists, and pushed off into the unknown. After gliding down the side of the multi-thousand-foot mountain, the 3 men – bruised and cut – were still a long way away from the whaling station. After 6 hours of marching – tired and in unknown territory – the men decided to take a nap. A 30-minute nap was agreed, and Shackleton watched over as his 2 men slept. After only 5 minutes he woke them and told them it had been 30 minutes. Continuing their march, eventually they noticed the water of Fortuna Bay, and further forward in their sights were the mountains of Stormness Bay. Another small victory, met with handshakes between the men. After the break of day, as the men sat and ate their breakfast, they heard a sound that they recognised as a whistle from the whaling station. The sound of encouragement! The sound of the outside world, finally. After another steep trek, met with many more obstacles, the men finally reached the whaling station, making their first contact with humanity in over a year and a half.

The very next morning, the 3 men that were left behind on the other end of the island were rescued. 3 days later, the men set off to return to Elephant Island, where they had left the rest of the crew. After 3 months, and 4 failed attempts, Shackleton finally saw the coast of Elephant Island.

August 30th, 1916, they returned to find that all 22 crew members had survived. Remarkable!

Living up to its name, the journey of this ship was one of endurance. Endurance by definition is the ability to withstand a difficult process without giving way. The journey of physical wellness is one that requires endurance – beyond physically. It is long, mentally challenging, and at times; it may even seem physically unbearable. What is required is pre-planning, grit, and determination. Although Shackleton and his men knew the journey wouldn't be straightforward, they had no idea what was actually waiting for them. They were forced to fight off leopard seals; and if they weren't strong enough, those seals would have killed, or at the very least, rocked the boat and caused them to drown.

A closer look.

On your wellness journey, people may attack you with pessimism, but you will need to be strong enough to not let this rock your boat and knock you into the sea of negativity. As for the dogs; let's think of them as a release, down-time. For example: having a night out, a cheat meal, a day off – these are your dogs. It is easy for our downtime to shift from relaxation to dependency over time – eventually making sacrifice more difficult – and most of the time, this may go unnoticed. When on our journey, rest is vital; as it gives our bodies and minds a chance to recharge – making long term discipline more sustainable. But what may start out as a necessary break, or a treat, can easily become a habit. In the story of Endurance, as the journey got more difficult over time, Shackleton and his men found a new purpose for the once sled-dogs. The dogs eventually became pets to the men; which made it more difficult to kill and eat them when the time called for it. If your cheat meal, your day off, and nights out, move away from their original purpose – downtime – and instead, become instruments of pleasure, it will undoubtedly be more difficult to kill them when needed. 1 cheat meal can easily turn into 2; just as a planned rest day can become a trigger to take more days off. To survive your voyage, you must be wary of your tools of recovery becoming pleasurable shortcuts to satisfaction. This is a crutch to your journey. Instead, you must be capable of sacrificing your dogs. Remember your overall goal, the initial purpose for the dogs, and do not look forward to the reward more than the journey itself. The reward is just a tool!

In their search for the whaling station, the men celebrated every victory; no matter how small. The completion of a small task is always a major contribution to the overall goal, and this is what you must remember. Yes, we have our plans – but we must not be rigid, and instead, show flexibility where needed. The men hadn't planned for the ship to be stuck in pack ice, but the decision had to be made to abandon ship and adjust their strategy in accordance with the obstacle. In our case, this may include changing a particular workout, or dietary approach, rather than sticking to something that clearly isn't working for us. Sometimes, a lifeboat (or 3) will come in handy.

Shackleton had a goal, and that goal was to cross the Antarctic continent. To do so, he knew he needed others on board to play a role. As the captain of your ship, it is your duty to make sure you keep the right people on board. From competent coaches to motivated training partners, and even friends who offer nothing more to your journey other than words of encouragement. This should never be overlooked. The good mood of Shackleton and his men was a significant factor in how they managed to endure many of their struggles. Whoever is aboard your ship, it is important that they align with your mission.

The Power of a Partner

There's hardly anything I find more pleasing than seeing couples working out together. The dynamics of a home are often determined by the tone set by those leading it – and in many households, that means the couple at the core.

I hadn't known many couples who exercised together. For most of the relationships I'd observed, it was usually one or the other who took fitness seriously. But I became curious: does working out together have any bearing on the strength of a relationship?

If we factor in the release of endorphins that comes with exercise, we might conclude that if both individuals in a relationship regular release endorphins, this could improve the overall mood within that unit – thus minimising stress levels.

Generally speaking, we gain satisfaction from being understood, especially by our partners. One way to foster that understanding – both giving and receiving – is by being on the same journey in more ways than one. A wellness journey is a powerful path to walk together.

Joint exercise among strangers builds a bond. So, it makes sense that exercise between friends – or lovers – strengthens their bond even more. Sharing a physical habit or lifestyle creates shared value in the relationship.

Now let's not pretend. For many of us, physical attraction toward our partner plays an important role. And studies show that exercise can trigger bodily responses similar to romantic stimulation.

In one study, adults were shown photos of the opposite sex before and after a 15-minute workout. When surveyed, they reported a higher level of attraction to the same images **after** the workout than they had **before.**

Why? Because adrenaline plays a key role in attraction – and adrenaline is released in larger quantities during exercise.

So, if physical attraction can be heightened through movement, two people in a relationship can absolutely benefit sexually and emotionally from exercising together. And couples who report higher levels of attraction for each other also tend to report having sex more frequently.

With all this in mind, we can safely assume that couples who work out together increase their satisfaction on multiple fronts.

Longevity and the Ones We Love

When it comes to living longer, your significant other – or your closest circle of loved ones – has an outsized influence. One of the strongest factors in this is **correspondence:** being encouraged, influenced, and inspired by those around you.

This isn't limited to romantic partnerships. It's a broader sentiment echoed by longevity researcher and author Dan Buettner, in his book "Live to 100: Secrets of the Blue Zones".

"Blue Zones" refer to regions in the world where people live significantly longer lives than average. These include:

- Okinawa, Japan
- Ikaria, Greece

- Nuoro Province, Sardinia (Italy)
- Nicoya Peninsula, Costa Rica
- Loma Linda, California
- Singapore

Buettner studied these areas and found they all shared the following key lifestyle factors:

- Community - Valuing family and maintaining strong social bonds, which leads to happiness and reduced cortisol levels.
- Movement – Daily, consistent movement, often out of necessity: walking, gardening, fishing, farming. In Blue Zones, a sedentary life is almost unthinkable.
- A primarily plant-based diet – Not necessarily vegetarian, but meat and animal products are consumed in moderation. Food is fresh, often homegrown, and minimally processed – contributing to its high standard. Olive oil is also preferred over other oils.
- Good sleep – Consistent, restful sleep aligned with natural circadian rhythms. Sleep isn't seen as optional – it's a priority that contributes to long, quality lives.

Living longer is one thing. Living well as you age – that's the real goal.

Being self-reliant and mobile, rather than dependent and static (with no shame to those who are), is often a more sustainable and fulfilling experience. And that outcome is directly shaped by the choices we make earlier in life.

V02 Max: The Oxygen Advantage

The oxygen your body takes in during exercise is measured by something called **V02 Max** – the maximum rate at which oxygen is adsorbed and used. And oxygen isn't just for staying alive – it is key to performing well when we exercise.

Here's why:

- ATP (adenosine triphosphate) is the energy that powers our muscles. Without this, the muscles will fail to operate properly.
- During exercise, ATP breaks down into ADP (adenosine diphosphate) to release energy and fuel muscle contractions.
- Oxygen is essential for producing more ATP.

In short, a higher V02 Max means better energy, performance, and endurance. But the benefits go even deeper.

Studies have found a positive correlation between V02 Max and reduced risk of both, disease-specific mortality and all-cause mortality. In other words, it can be used as a predictor of how long – and how well – you will live.

While V02 Max naturally declines with age, maintaining an optimal level for your age offers protection from various cardiovascular diseases.

You can improve V02 Max through:

- Running
- Cycling
- Rowing
- Swimming
- Interval training
- Brisk walking

These are all recommended by doctors for healthy aging.

Laying the Groundwork While You're Young

Exercising in your youth doesn't just benefit you in the present – it sets you up for the future.

Some of the long-term benefits include:

1. Weight management

This isn't about losing fat. Resistance training and weightlifting help preserve muscle mass, which is crucial as we age. After 50, we typically lose one-third of our muscle mass. By 70, the rate of loss increases even more.

Loss of muscle leads to:

- Fatigue
- Higher risk of fractures
- Increased dependence on others
- Decreased mobility

2. Cognitive Function

Exercise has been shown to improve brain structure and boost memory. The hippocampus – the part of the brain responsible for memory – increases in volume with consistent physical activity.

- Sedentary lifestyles are linked to Alzheimer's.
- Exercise reduces dementia risk by up to 30%.
- Alzheimer's disease risk alone is cut by 45% with regular activity.

With over 55 million people worldwide suffering from dementia, and a projected 100% increase every 20 years, the stakes are high.

The One Exercise I Must Recommend

I'd feel guilty if I didn't recommend this form of movement -- **hill sprints.**

Despite requiring no equipment, hill sprints have been likened to weight training because of the full-body benefits they offer.

- Build muscle
- Enhance running power
- Improve cardiovascular health
- Torch fat through metabolic stimulation

Hill sprints engage nearly every muscle in the body while training both the anaerobic and aerobic energy systems. Due to the uphill motion, you contact the ground sooner, which limits your range of motion and reduces impact. Sprinting uphill also provides us with a resistance that impairs our ability to use maximum force (despite using maximum effort), and this reduces the risk of injury.

This is a great exercise to adopt in your younger years – you'll feel the benefits well into later life. While hill sprints aren't essential in older age, many people still incorporate them in their fitness routine. What does remain essential in older age are mobility exercises.

Improved mobility leads to:

- Better posture
- Reduced muscle tension
- Easier breathing
- Better digestion
- More energy
- Lower risk of injury

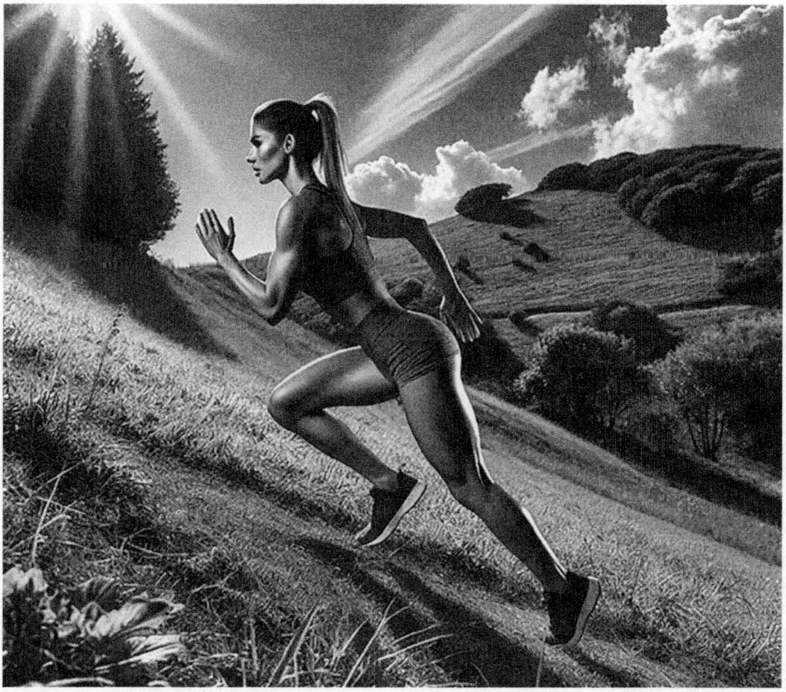

Simple mobility exercises for older adults include:

- Squats
- Wall push-ups
- Resistance band workouts
- Hip stretches
- Bridges
- Sit-to-stand exercises
- Spinal twists

If self-motivation is hard, or hiring a personal trainer isn't an option, consider joining a yoga or Pilates class. Alternatively, if you're not keen on a group environment, you can find an online channel for guided movement at home. But if the group setting energises you, seek out local walking or running clubs. Not only do they keep you active – they also offer the community vibe we see in every Blue Zone. There is something for every'body'.

Let Inspiration Move You

Let people like Elaine Lalane remind us of what's possible. At 98 years old – at the time of this books release – she still does full body workouts.

Yes, genetics can play a part. But don't be mistaken, lifestyle is the main character in the story of longevity.

So whether it's your partner, your community, or your inner voice calling – you owe it to yourself to move.

Not later.

Not when it's convenient.

Not when you feel like it.

Move **now** – and keep moving.

Because every rep is a declaration:

That you love yourself.

That you choose vitality.

That you believe in a longer, fuller, better life.
Together, or alone, you've got this.
Just move.

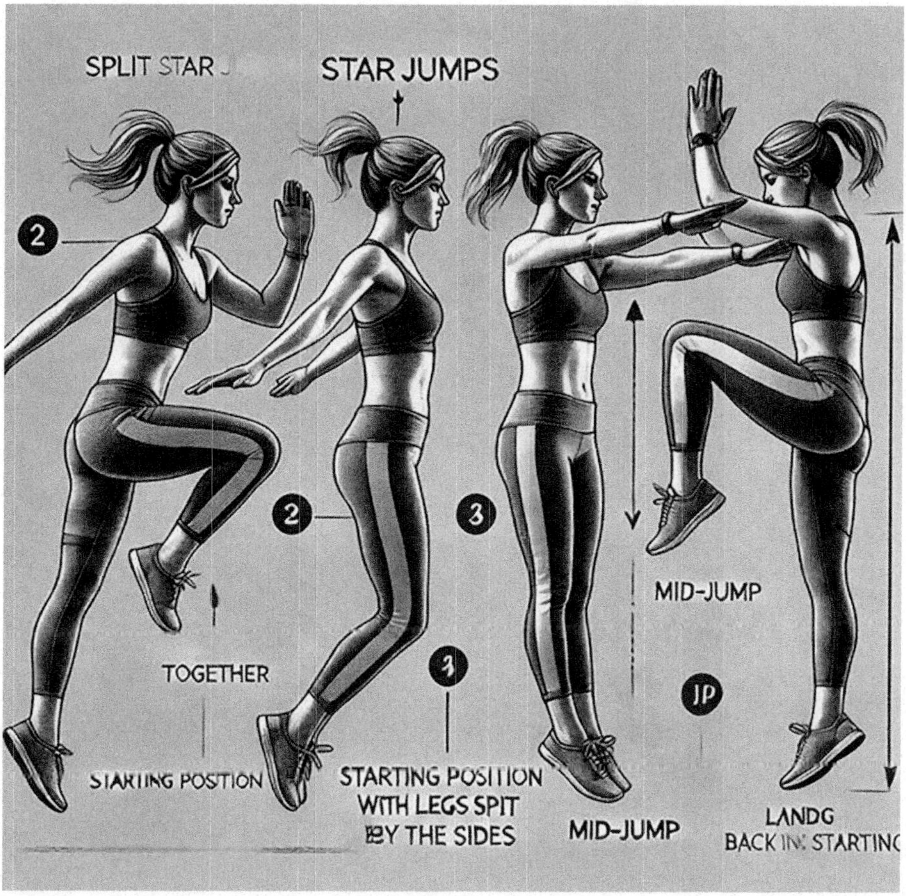

CHAPTER 10

The power of hope.

What I love most about the pursuit of wellness is that you only fail when you stop chasing it. As long as you keep moving forward, you're still in the game. Wellness is a journey of continuity. It is not a process; because processes have an end. This journey becomes a lifestyle.

We shouldn't be discouraged when the results we see in the moment don't match our expectations. A pothole isn't the end of the road, and a hurdle is not the finish line. Persistence breaks resistance.

The way we approach our smaller goals translates directly into how we tackle larger ones. An exercise-based goal may seem "small," not because it's easy, but because it's something entirely within your control.

You are stronger than the limits your mindset tries to impose. Most of us underestimate ourselves, placing irrational ceilings on our dreams. (See section on autosuggestion.) Sometimes, these limitations are inherited – passed down from well-meaning parents, teachers, or mentors who, without realising it, taught us to fear failure more than to chase possibility. We tend to absorb the doubts of those around us. And often, those doubts quietly become our beliefs.

This is the essence of self-fulfilling prophecy: our expectations dictate our outcome.

That's why it's so important to surround yourself with people who are either in – or moving toward – the position you strive for. Positive examples are infectious. Environment matters. Shape one that aligns with your goals and watch how quickly things begin to shift. When you believe in the destination, your plan will be executed with confidence.

Consider the story of Roger Bannister.

On May 6th, 1954, Bannister – a medical student at the time – did what the world had deemed impossible: he ran a mile in under four minutes. For decades, breaking the four-minute mile had been discussed, attempted, and failed. Experts believed it to be physiologically unattainable. The theory was that the human heart and lungs simply couldn't supply the muscles with enough oxygen to maintain the required speed.

In 1952, Bannister narrowly missed an Olympic medal. In 1953, he ran the mile in 4:04 – agonisingly close to the barrier. Others came close as well. But instead of accepting the limit, Bannister studied it. Trained for it. Strategised for it. And in 1954, he broke it – not in perfect conditions, but in cold, wet weather. Even experts had said those conditions wouldn't be favourable. He'd planned his race with precision, knowing exactly when and how to pace himself for a strong finish.

Here's what's fascinating: just 46 days after Bannister's historic race, another runner broke the same barrier. A year later, three more men broke it – in the same race. Today, nearly 2,000 runners have recorded a mile in under four minutes.

What changed?

Not human physiology. Human belief.

The barrier was never physical – it was mental. Once people **saw** it could be done, they **knew** it could be done. Representation replaced limitation.

Bannister's self-belief created a new reality not only for himself, but for everyone watching.

This is why mindset matters. Belief alone isn't enough – Bannister also had a plan. But without belief, the plan wouldn't have mattered.

The takeaway is this: physical attainment is never just physical. It starts in the mind. Once belief enters, change follows.

Words are the medicine.

Jennifer; a proud mother from the countryside of Jamaica, once said to her young son:

"You are in charge of your results".

At the time he was struggling as an aspiring athlete. But those words stuck. They played in the back of his mind for years to come. Today, that boy is a man who's become one of the most iconic athletes in history. He says much of his drive and determination came from what he was told as a child.

"From an early age they always said to me: son don't let nobody put you in a box. Work hard and live your dreams"

- Usain Bolt, 8-time Olympic gold medalist.

Words can plant seeds. But what we do with those words – how we live them out – is what produces the fruit.

Say it. Plan it. Do it.

Lawrence Okolie, once an obese teenager working in McDonald's, made the decision to change his life. While on his lunch break, he watched Olympic boxing on TV – and something clicked.

Inspired, he walked up to his manager and said he'd be cutting back his hours. He wanted to train full-time to become a boxer. Years later, he would become a world champion.

Okolie admitted that he wasn't the most naturally disciplined person. But a shift in **mentality** changed everything. He spoke his goal, created a plan, and stuck to it. And that changed the course of his life.

Mind. Body. Mind

At 17, American psychiatrist Milton H. Erickson was diagnosed with polio and left paralysed. Doctors told him he would never walk again. But through deep meditation and focused mental effort, he defied the odds and learned how to move.

While confined to his bed, he began observing people closely – developing an uncanny understanding of human behaviour. Later in life, this insight shaped his approach to therapy.

One of his patients struggled with overeating, smoking, and drinking. Instead of demanding the patient quit everything at once, Erickson designed a plan that required movement. The patient had to walk three blocks for every meal – so food had to be earned. He could still drink, but only one drink per bar – requiring barhopping on foot. Cigarettes were allowed too, but the matches were kept downstairs and the cigarettes upstairs.

It wasn't punishment – it was intention.

Erickson knew that changing the **way** we move can change the **way** we think. He believed movement was stimulation, and that without stimulation, we often turn to destructive habits to feel **something.**

And he was right.

Hope Molecules

When we exercise, our muscles release small proteins called **myokines** into the bloodstream. These are nicknamed "hope molecules" for good reason – they've been shown to have antidepressant effects.

Simple movements like walking or cycling can trigger the release of these chemicals. This is why something as small as a brisk morning walk can dramatically shift our mood and mindset.

Even in the corporate world, leaders are starting to catch on. "Walking meetings" and treadmill brainstorming sessions are becoming popular – because movement fuels creativity, clarity, and connection.

The Heavyweight Mindset

"Exercise gets you out of a bad place"
– Tyson Fury, former World Heavyweight Champion.

Fury, who lives with bipolar disorder and depression, credits regular exercise with keeping him grounded. He's said that if he skips two days of training, the fog of depression begins to creep back in.

Exercise isn't just about health. It's about survival. Physical activity is as essential to our being as eating and breathing. Yet many of us have drifted far from that truth.

But with the right knowledge – and consistent action – we can reconnect with our instinct to move. And when we do, the benefits extend far beyond our bodies.

Your Best Friend

Let's take a moment to personify exercise. Imagine exercise as a human – a dynamic and multifaceted character. Let's call this character **Caelius.**

Caelius is complex, with many roles and expressions. Because of its characteristics, Caelius can be highly influential.

Born from necessity, Caelius is instinctive and innocent in intention. Despite not always being the friend we want, Caelius is the friend we all need.

Take my friend Sharon, for example. As a teenager, Sharon's home life was turbulent, with her parents often arguing in front of her. One day, after hearing about the benefits involved, Sharon decided to befriend Caelius. Whenever her parents argued, Caelius showed up, offering her an escape. To this day, Sharon credits her best friend Caelius for bringing her peace in times of chaos.

Caelius is more than just a friend when we need an escape. Caelius is a healer, preserving our bodies. A strict parent, teaching discipline and organisation. A teacher, fostering teamwork. A motivator, building confidence. A guru, helping us discover who we truly are.

But Caelius is neutral – neither inherently good nor bad. It's up to us how we choose to use this character. Guided with care, Caelius becomes a vessel for transformation. Misused, Caelius can take on a darker role, punishing rather than empowering.

Caelius has a place in all our lives. This book is your guide to building the strongest, most rewarding relationship with Caelius – a relationship that transforms not just your body, but your mind and character as well. Together, we'll unlock the potential of this powerful companion and learn to use it in ways that serve both ourselves and the world around us.

Just like you

Over the years, I've worked with people from all walks of life. And I always ask them the same question:

What drives you to work-out? How does it make your life better?

Here's what they had to say:

"When I exercise, I feel good about myself. Because of that feeling, my confidence is boosted, and I'm able to express that in other areas of my life. I've found that my chances of success within these other areas increase – because I approach life with belief. It's the initial feel-good approach that transcends everything!"
- Jonathan Shaer

"It makes me feel good knowing I'm doing something for my body. I get peace of mind knowing I'm doing all that I can to live longer."
- J.T

"Transferable confidence! I feel that I can physically look after myself now, and that's made me stand up for myself more in life too. That all comes from the training."
- Carl Thornton

"All of the burdens I take on from other people – it can get overwhelming. But when I do boxing training, it's like an escape. No matter how difficult the session is, I always feel a sense of relief."
- David Tugendhaft

"It's a release. After a long day of work, my focus shifts completely to the workout. Whatever stresses I have in the outside world fades away."
- S.W

"I always prefer when the sessions are difficult. Because when I finish them, I have the belief that I'm capable of more than I thought. I take that same belief into my daily life."
- Zahra

"It sets the tone for my day before I start work. It's like a wake-up call. But I also get the feeling of accomplishment from it – and that's how I like to live."
- Joseph H

The final words

What began with watching "Rocky" and doing push-ups in my bedroom has become something much bigger than me. I've trained athletes, everyday people, and those who never thought they'd fall in love with movement – but did. And through all of them, I've seen the same truth reflected back:

We were never just training our bodies. We were always training our character.

Exercise isn't just a way to build strength. It's how we learn discipline, face our fears, manage failure, and chase something better – day after day. When you show up for your body, you show up for your life.

You've read the stories. You've seen how history, biology, and the human spirit all point toward one thing: we are made to move. But more importantly, we are made to grow. And growth demands effort. Effort demands action – and action starts with a choice.

Movement changes your mind.
A changed mind changes your life.
And that changed life can change others.

Absorb the lessons.
Apply the lessons.
Share the lessons.

You already have everything you need.
Now move.

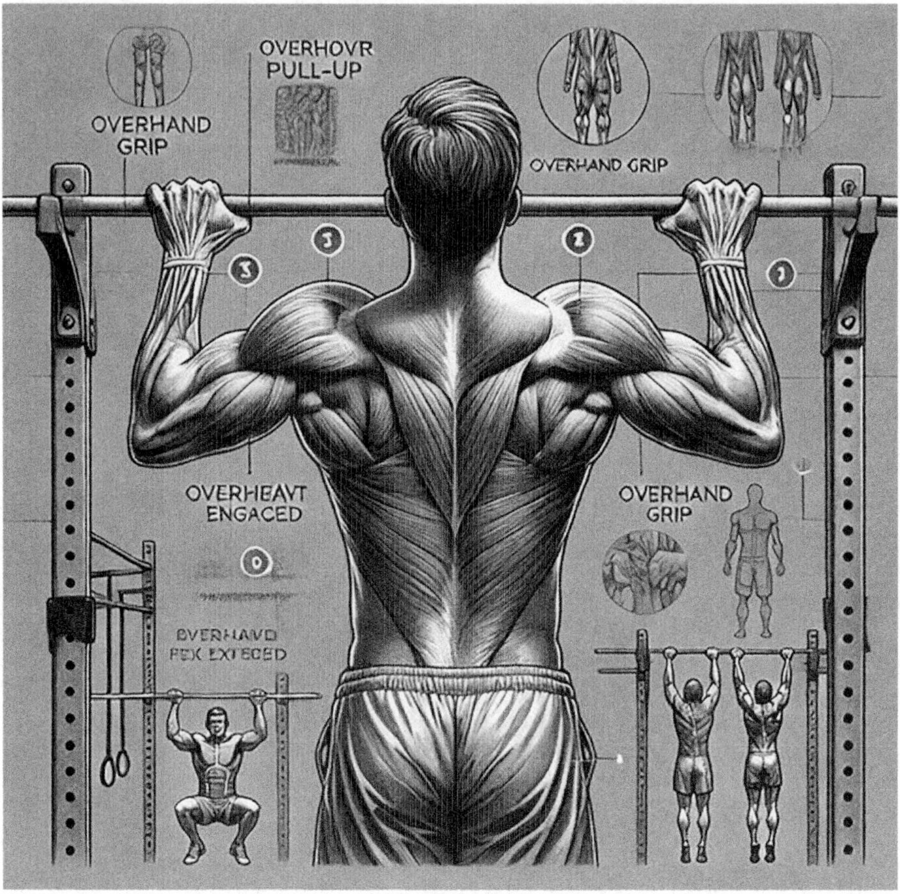
OVERHAND
GRIP
OVERHOVR
PULL-UP
OVERHAND GRIP
OVERHEAVT
ENGACED
OVERHAND
GRIP

Bibliography

Books:

• Duhigg, C. (2012). The Power of Habit: Why We Do What We Do in Life and Business. Random House.
• Justice, G. (2016). Pride & Discipline: The Legacy of Jack LaLanne. Greg Justice Publishing.
• Nardi, D. (2011). Neuroscience of Personality: Brain Savvy Insights for All Types of People. Radiance House.
• Robbins, J. (2000). A Symphony in the Brain: The Evolution of the New Brainwave Biofeedback. Grove Press.
• Greene, R. (2018). The Laws of Human Nature. Viking.
Van der Kolk, Bessel A. The Body Keeps the Score: Brain, Mind, and Body in the Healing of Trauma. New York: Viking, 2014.

Articles and Websites:

• Chattjee, R. (2018). "Where Did Agriculture Begin? Oh Boy, It's Complicated." PRI's The World. Retrieved from https://www.pri.org.
• Dalleck, L. C. (n.d.). The History of Fitness. Retrieved from PositivePsychology.com.
• McCluskey, M. (n.d.). "The Triumph of Women in Sparta." The Conversation. Keele University. Retrieved from https://theconversation.com.
• Naples, M. (2018). "The Triumphant Women of Sparta." Ancient Origins. Retrieved from https://ancient-origins.net.
• "Charmion: Natty Life – Bodybuilding History." (n.d.). YouTube. Retrieved from https://www.youtube.com.

• "Elaine LaLanne, A Life in Fitness." (2023). The New York Times. Retrieved from https://www.nytimes.com.
• "Cerebellar Stroke Recovery." (n.d.). Flint Rehab. Retrieved from https://www.flintrehab.com.
• "Louis van Gaal's Tactical Philosophy." (2014). Defending With the Ball Blog. Retrieved from https://defendingwiththeball.wordpress.com.
• Bridge, F. (n.d.). "Frankie Bridge on Exercise and Anxiety." Women's Fitness. Retrieved from https://womensfitness.co.uk.

Journals and Academic Sources:

• National Center for Biotechnology Information (n.d.). Retrieved from https://ncbi.nlm.nih.gov.
• University College London (n.d.). Retrieved from https://ucl.ac.uk.
• Purdue University (n.d.). Retrieved from https://purdue.edu.

Additional Sources:

• "Usain Bolt's Career and Legacy." (n.d.). Essentially Sports. Retrieved from https://essentiallysports.com.
• Runner's World. (n.d.). Retrieved from https://runnersworld.com.
• NLPCourses.com. (n.d.). Retrieved from https://nlpcourses.com.
• "Silhouettes: The Eras We Build (1899–1914)." (n.d.). Silhouettes Costumes. Retrieved from https://silhouettescostumes.com.
• This is Africa. (n.d.). Retrieved from https://thisisafrica.me.
• Politics.co.uk. (n.d.). Retrieved from https://politics.co.uk.

Printed in Dunstable, United Kingdom

72031486R00080